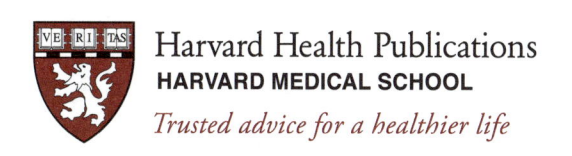

Harvard Health Publications
HARVARD MEDICAL SCHOOL
Trusted advice for a healthier life

Dear Reader,

The numbers are shocking. Just three out 10 American adults are active enough to stay healthy and fit. Nearly four out of 10 admit they aren't active at all, despite reams of research proving that exercise is a powerful preventive, and sometimes an antidote, for disability and illness. Which side of this divide are you standing on—and why?

Maybe you're not sure what blend of exercise is best. Or perhaps you know exactly what you need to do, but your workouts have become so halfhearted and humdrum that it's harder than ever to dig up the energy to do them. Do you want to jump-start your sputtering exercise program? Or are you stuck on a plateau and wishing you could kick it up to the next level?

This special report is just the ticket. This collaboration brings together the experience we've each gained in our respective fields of physical medicine and rehabilitation as well as personal training. The nine workouts inside will challenge your body and spirit in a variety of ways while warding off boredom. You can switch up workouts before your motivation tanks, or work hard on mastering a few. Further, we've designed the exercises so that you can tailor each one to your fitness level. Is an exercise too hard? Try the easier option. Too easy? Step up the challenge.

We've laid out the tools you need to take charge in this report, which is packed with up-to-the-moment news you can use on exercise. So go ahead. Set your goals. Check our safety tips. Select one or more workouts you'd like to master. And mix it up every month to six weeks to stay motivated. Your body—and mind—will thank you.

Sincerely,

Edward Phillips, MD

Edward M. Phillips, M.D.
Medical Editor

Josie Gardiner   *Joy Prouty*

Josie Gardiner and Joy Prouty
Master Trainers and Fitness Consultants

Special thanks to the Equinox fitness club on Dartmouth Street in Boston for the use of its facilities, and to the following Equinox personal trainers, instructors, and staff members for demonstrating the exercises depicted in this report: Peter Athans, Maryanne Blake, Kristy DiScipio, Josie Gardiner, Shane Genakos, and Albert Roberson.

Harvard Health Publications | Harvard Medical School | 10 Shattuck Street, Second Floor | Boston, MA 02115

Diving in

Let's get right to the point: why exercise? The pleasing image of smooth, well-defined muscles and a slimmer silhouette prods many people into activity. But in the long run, more robust health and enhanced prospects for joyful, full-tilt living at every age may provide even deeper, more satisfying rewards.

Picking up this report is the first step. From warming up to cooling down and everything in between, we'll show you exercises to work out all the major muscle groups, whether you're at the gym, at home, or traveling. There are plenty of options here, so you can change your routine whenever you grow bored with it or it becomes too easy. But in the meantime, in case you're tempted to slack off, this section provides plenty of reasons to lace up your gym shoes and get moving.

Why work your body?

If you're like most people, you have a lot of demands on your time, so finding the opportunity to exercise may take some planning. Yet regular physical activity makes an enormous difference to the quality and length of your life, a fact underscored by hundreds of solid studies. Here are some of the findings from those studies—with plenty of reasons to get moving:

- Exercise can add years to your life. In the long-running Framingham Heart Study, moderate activity tacked on 1.3 years of life for men and 1.5 years of life for women when compared with low activity. Raising the bar to high activity added 3.7 years for men and 3.5 years for women.
- Exercise lessens your risk of heart disease, the No. 1 killer of Americans. It does this in several ways. For example, exercising regularly helps prevent plaque buildup by striking a healthier balance of blood lipids (HDL, LDL, and triglycerides), and it helps arteries retain resilience despite the effects of aging. Even if you already have heart disease, exercise lowers your chances of dying from it.
- Exercise also lowers blood pressure, a boon for many body systems. Long-term high blood pressure (hypertension) doubles or triples the odds of developing heart failure and often paves the path to other kinds of heart disease, stroke, aortic aneurysm, and kidney disease or failure.
- Exercise can help prevent diabetes by paring off excess weight, modestly lowering blood sugar levels, and boosting sensitivity to insulin so your body needs less of it. If you already have diabetes, exercise helps control blood sugar.
- Exercise reduces the risk for developing cancers of the colon, breast, endometrium (uterine lining), and prostate. By helping you maintain a healthy weight, exercise also lessens your risk for other cancers in which obesity is a factor.
- Exercise helps shore up bones, which reach peak density and strength during the first three decades of life. Over time, bones become lacier and weaker as density slips away. Weight-bearing exercises like running and strength training, when combined with calcium, vitamin D, and bone-saving medications if necessary, help ward off bone loss. And balance-enhancing activities, including tai chi and

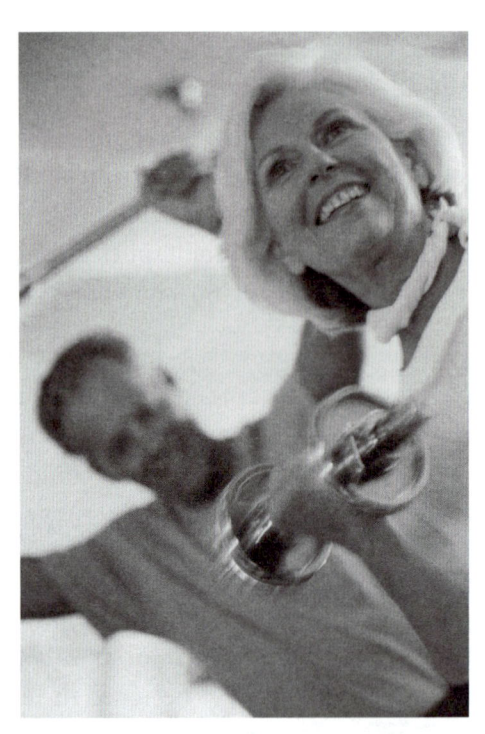

yoga, help prevent falls that may end in fractures.
- Exercise helps protect joints by easing swelling, pain, and fatigue and by keeping cartilage healthy. Strong muscles support joints and lighten the load on them. Activities that boost flexibility, such as stretching, yoga, and tai chi, extend range of motion.
- Exercise may limit or even reverse knee or hip pain by helping to control weight—a big deal, since every added pound multiplies knee stress fourfold, according to the Arthritis Foundation.
- Exercise can lift spirits by releasing mood-elevating neurotransmitters, relieving stress, and promoting a sense of well-being. In some studies, regular exercise eased mild to moderate depression as effectively as medications. Combining exercise with medications, therapy, and social engagement is even better.
- Exercise reduces insomnia and improves overall sleep quality. Exercise is the only proven way to increase the amount of time you spend in deep sleep, the type that particularly restores your energy. Moreover, adequate sleep lowers your risks of developing heart disease, type 2 diabetes, and even dementia.
- Exercise may improve obstructive sleep apnea. In a recent analysis of five studies, a structured exercise program helped reduce the severity of sleep apnea, even in the absence of significant weight loss.
- Exercise could even boost your ability to fend off infection. Three randomized trials of women who walked briskly 35 to 45 minutes a day, five days a week for 12 to 15 weeks, found that these women experienced half the cold symptoms of a sedentary group. Additional research shows exercise prompts a modest, short-term upswing in natural killer cells and white blood cells, which help squelch infection.

How much time should you spend on exercise?

Text messages dinging, emails thudding into your inbox, cellphone and work phone simultaneously ringing. Some days, it's hard to find a moment to think, let alone shoehorn in a visit to the gym or even a quick walk.

Fortunately, just 30 minutes of moderately intense aerobic activity five days a week (a total of 150 minutes a week) delivers solid health benefits, according to the Physical Activity Guidelines for Americans from the U.S. Department of Health and Human Services. You don't have to do all 30 minutes in a single daily session. For example, you can reach these goals by performing chunks of daily exercise in 10-minute blocks. (Alternately, you can achieve the same results with vigorous aerobic activity in half the time—a total of 75 minutes a week—or you can do an equivalent mix of moderate and vigorous exercise. For examples of moderate versus vigorous types of activity, go to

Work your mind

Want to stay mentally sharp? Stay active! Even mild activity boosts blood flow to the brain—and, in turn, the vital oxygenation that keeps neural networks humming.

Exercise also boosts mental performance by improving sleep quality and reducing insomnia. Learning, memory, and the ability to solve puzzles are all enhanced by a good night's rest. In a systematic review, exercise training was shown to improve sleep quality in middle-aged and older adults.

Moreover, a Mayo Clinic review confirmed that exercise significantly reduces the risk of problems with thinking, memory, and even dementia as a person ages and should be included as a prescription for protecting brain health. Studies have shown less age-related shrinkage of brain tissue in physically fit participants ages 55 to 79 and sharper executive control functions, such as attention, organization, and planning, among exercisers ages 55 to 80.

Physical activity may even stimulate the growth of brain cells. This regeneration—or plasticity, as neurologists call it—may help the nervous system combat some effects of aging or conditions like stroke that injure the brain.

Finally, regular exercise helps prevent or reduce other health problems that harm the brain, such as

- high blood pressure and elevated lipids that contribute to artery-clogging atherosclerosis, which reduces the flow of oxygen to brain cells
- diabetes, which can compromise memory
- transient ischemic attacks ("mini-strokes," in which blood flow to the brain is briefly interrupted) or full-fledged strokes that can destroy swaths of brain cells.

www.health.harvard.edu/activities.) If you're able to double the time you spend exercising, the guidelines indicate that five hours (300 minutes) of moderate aerobic activity a week will give you more extensive health benefits.

In addition to aerobic work, the experts also recommend twice-weekly strength training sessions for all major muscle groups, and balance exercises for older adults at risk of falling.

Stand up for your health

Structured workouts like the ones in this report are essential for optimal health. But you should also try to stand and move around more during the day, especially if you have a desk job. Sitting for hours on end can increase your risk of serious ailments such as heart disease, type 2 diabetes, and certain cancers. By contrast, you can lower your risks of all of these conditions simply by standing and moving more—even if you already exercise. That's because routine movement during the day adds on to those benefits.

That was the conclusion of a large, long-term study of 123,000 middle-aged adults by researchers from the American Cancer Society, published in the *American Journal of Epidemiology*. Women who sat the most had a 34% greater risk of dying from any cause over the 14 years of the study compared with those who sat the least. For men, the increase was 17%. When exercise was factored in, the difference was even more stark. The most sedentary women, who neither moved nor exercised a lot, were almost twice as likely to die as those who moved and exercised the most. The most sedentary men were 50% more likely to die than their more active counterparts. Similarly, other studies have concluded that routine, everyday movement has benefits, whether for heart disease, diabetes, cancer, or weight loss. It's gotten to the point now where some doctors actually advise their patients to use sitting "in moderation."

Why does prolonged sitting have such negative health consequences? One explanation is that it relaxes your largest muscles. When muscles relax, they take up very little sugar (glucose) from the blood, upping your risk of type 2 diabetes. In addition, the enzymes that break down blood fats (triglycerides) plummet, causing levels of the "good" cholesterol, HDL, to fall, too. The result is a higher risk of heart disease.

By contrast, everyday movement not only reduces your risk of major ailments, but also helps you burn more calories. Dr. James Levine at the Mayo Clinic coined the term "non-exercise activity thermogenesis," or NEAT, to refer to the energy you burn through ordinary activity that you don't think of as exercise, such as fidgeting, carrying the laundry upstairs, dancing around the house to your favorite tune, or even standing while you talk on the phone. In one study, he measured NEAT in lean and obese people, all of whom had similar jobs and were forbidden to exercise during the course of the study. There was one key difference between the two groups. The obese people sat longer than their lean counterparts, by an average of two-and-a-half hours more per day.

Setting goals and motivating yourself

What are your goals and motivation for working out? It's obvious that exercise is essential to your health. But it could help to set your eyes on another prize, too—maybe cruising across the finish line of a 10K race or just slipping into a favorite pair of jeans. Setting exercise goals can change idle hopes into reality, especially if you put some supports in place.

Slimming down

Losing weight hinges on simple math. Taking in more calories than you burn adds pounds; burning off more calories than you take in shaves off pounds. A moderately active person who gets about 30 minutes of exercise a day needs 15 calories of food to maintain each pound of his or her body weight. To lose a pound a week, you need to lop off about 500 calories a day by eating less and adding on activity time.

If weight loss is your goal, step up to 60 minutes of moderate to vigorous activity at least five days a week. Depending on your body type, however, you may need 60 to 90 minutes a day of moderate activity to drop pounds and keep them off.

How can you manage this? First, understand that the exercises described in our workouts are just one slice of physical activity. So invest chunks of time in performing the workouts in this report, but also expect to tack on time spent walking briskly or burning calories through other activities. If you want to know how many calories specific activities chomp up, check www.health.harvard.edu/burncalories.

Carrot or stick?

Motivation takes many forms, so pick the carrot or stick that works for you. Maybe you'd like to tune your muscles to tackle new activities, like climbing a towering

Just how fit are you?

Remember running laps and crunching out sit-ups on the dusty mats of your elementary school gym as a stopwatch ticked away? That's not just for kids anymore, now that the President's Council on Fitness, Sports, and Nutrition has recast the Youth Fitness Test with adults in mind. Click on www.adultfitnesstest.org to see how you fare in simple tests of aerobic fitness, strength, flexibility, and body composition.

rock wall, churning through the water during a triathlon, or powering up Heartbreak Hill on the heels of elite runners in the Boston Marathon. Perhaps you hope to be inching ever closer to a body you'd love to show off. Maybe you long for guiltless licks off an ice cream cone.

Perhaps a small bet with a friend—loser pays for kayaking lessons—or just wanting to hold up your end of the bargain with a new exercise partner will do the trick. To choose the best tack to take, start by filling out the "Planning worksheet" on page 6.

Setting your goals

A written record of your goals is a good reminder when life intrudes and interest flags. So copy the worksheet and put it where it can act as a daily nudge.

Finding support helps. Hiring a personal trainer or tapping a buddy for workouts or walks can supply motivation. Friends who can cheer you on and hold you accountable to your plan help, too. And most of us enjoy a reward, so write down pleasurable options if you meet weekly or daily goals. (Avoid food rewards or keep them small, lest they scrub out any benefits gained through exercise.) One reward is simply seeing progress, so consider measuring your gains at regular intervals (see "Measuring gains," page 11).

Planning worksheet

My goals are to

❏ enhance my health

❏ tone my muscles

❏ extend my endurance

❏ lose ____ pounds (a pound a week is reasonable, so break down bigger goals into smaller, manageable chunks) in the next ____ weeks

❏ strengthen my upper body

❏ strengthen my lower body

❏ strengthen my core and back muscles

❏ step up my game in a sport, such as _____ _____ _____

❏ be able to enjoy _____ _____ _____

(Here consider what tasks and fun you are missing out on. Does your back hurt? Are you finding it hard to climb stairs, smash an overhead in tennis, or dig deep while gardening?)

Right now, I exercise

❏ rarely or never

❏ once a week for _____ minutes

❏ twice a week for _____ minutes

❏ three to five times a week for _____ minutes

I'd like to

❏ exercise _____ times a week for _____ minutes

❏ add cardio exercise to my weekly routine

❏ add strength training to my weekly routine

❏ change up my weekly routine

My new plan:

Fill in some goals for a week, writing in cardio sessions like 30 minutes of brisk walking (remember, this can be in two or three chunks) or the workouts in this report that you plan to try. If you're wondering what mix of exercise to choose, read pages 7–9 and see Table 2 on page 17.

I can do

❏ _____ on Monday at _____

❏ _____ on Tuesday at _____

❏ _____ on Wednesday at _____

❏ _____ on Thursday at _____

❏ _____ on Friday at _____

❏ _____ on Saturday at _____

❏ _____ on Sunday at _____

I will gain support for my new plan by

❏ hiring a personal trainer on these days
   ❏ Monday ❏ Tuesday ❏ Wednesday
   ❏ Thursday ❏ Friday ❏ Saturday ❏ Sunday

❏ lining up an exercise partner for walks or workouts on these days
   ❏ Monday ❏ Tuesday ❏ Wednesday
   ❏ Thursday ❏ Friday ❏ Saturday ❏ Sunday

❏ telling a friend about my plan and asking him or her to check in with me once a week on _____ to cheer me on and encourage me to stay the course

❏ rewarding myself by doing _____ _____
   at the end of the week

❏ measuring my gains (see page 11) on _____

SPECIAL SECTION

Exercise 101

First, let's define some terms. Although the words "physical activity" and "exercise" are frequently swapped, they are not interchangeable. Physical activity refers to any movement you make that triggers muscle contractions and a rise in metabolism. This could include everyday activities such as housework or raking leaves. All physical activity is beneficial (see "Stand up for your health," page 4). But exercise is a structured program of activity to help you become physically fit.

Those aren't the only terms that can cause confusion. At your gym and even in this report, you may hear unfamiliar terms being tossed about. Check our explanations below and see how these concepts fit into the workouts.

Five components of fitness

All-around fitness calls for several types of activities. Generally, experts recommend a combination of aerobic activities and flexibility, strength, and balance exercises. One form of activity—relaxation—often gets short shrift, though it shouldn't. Relaxation helps ease health-busting stress.

1 Aerobic activities

Often called cardio or endurance activities, aerobic activities are great for burning calories and paring down unwanted fat. These activities—think of walking, biking, running, and swimming—push large muscles to repeatedly contract and relax. This temporarily boosts your heart rate and breathing, allowing more oxygen to reach your muscles and tuning up cardiovascular endurance.

Experts once believed cardio activities were beneficial only if you kept your heart rate hammering in the aerobic range—70% to 85% of your maximum heart rate—for a specified length of time. (Maximum heart rate is roughly estimated as 220 minus your age.) But research

Move a muscle

Muscle is tethered to bone by cords of tissue called tendons. A single muscle can contain 10,000 to more than a million muscle fibers, packed in numerous neat bundles and swathed in connective tissue known as the epimysium. Groups of muscle fibers receive marching instructions from a single nerve cell called a motor neuron. Together, this combination of nerve cell and muscle fibers constitutes one motor unit. The more fibers a nerve cell commands, the greater the force that motor unit exerts.

Most skeletal muscles have fast-twitch and slow-twitch fibers. Usually, both are pressed into service when you exercise. Slow-twitch fibers work best during low-intensity activities, which allow a good supply of oxygen. They get called on first for most activities and can keep acting for long periods. Fast-twitch fibers step into the breach to create bursts of power during high-intensity anaerobic activities. They supply more force, but are more quickly exhausted.

When nerve impulses originating in the brain shoot along neural pathways toward a muscle, they trigger a complex set of chemical reactions that cause muscle proteins called myofilaments to slide over each other, generating force. Movement occurs when that force ripples through the muscle structure to the tendons, which in turn tug on the bones. Essentially, the bunching muscles act like strings that make a puppet spring to life.

SPECIAL SECTION | Exercise 101

now shows you're gaining benefits even when working at a more moderate intensity.

How often to perform: The Physical Activity Guidelines for Americans recommend at least 150 minutes of moderate-intensity physical activity (such as a brisk walk) or 75 minutes of vigorous-intensity physical activity per week. You can also perform an equivalent combination of the two intensities. To judge the intensity of your workout, use our "How hard are you working?" chart (see Table 1, below right). As you start to work out more often, you'll notice gains as exercises become easier.

2 Strength training

Strength or resistance training, which typically uses equipment such as weight machines, free weights, and resistance bands or tubing, protects against bone loss and builds muscle. Technically, strength or resistance training takes place any time your muscles face a stronger-than-usual counterforce.

Isotonic actions, such as lifting a dumbbell from knee height to shoulder height, prompt muscles to shorten or lengthen to move the attached joint through its range of motion. The resistance the muscle works against—the dumbbell—is uniform.

Isometric actions, such as pushing against a wall or struggling to lift an extremely heavy weight, force muscles to work against fixed resistance, so no such shortening or lengthening occurs. In fact, there's no muscle movement, and resistance can vary depending on how hard you push against the wall or pull on the weight. While isometrics are a quick way to build muscle strength within a very limited range of motion, they're also the most stressful for your heart and circulatory system. You can safely build muscle strength and endurance through isotonic exercise without overtaxing your cardiovascular system.

Strength training with progressively heavier weights or increasing resistance makes muscles bigger—though usually not by much unless genetics allow this and you frequently perform challenging workouts. Even without obvious muscle growth, though, these activities enhance the ability of the nervous system to activate motor units (see "Move a muscle," page 7). Aside from toning you, strength training guarantees you'll have the functional strength to carry out everyday activities—lifting groceries, climbing stairs, rushing for the bus—with ease.

How often to perform: The Physical Activity Guidelines for Americans recommend two sessions a week. But note that your body needs *at least 48 hours* for recovery and repairs between strength training sessions (see "6 tips for effective strength training," page 16). So if you do an upper-body

Table 1: How hard are you working?

INTENSITY	IT FEELS…	YOU ARE…
Light	Easy	• Breathing easily • Warming up, but not yet sweating • Able to talk—or even sing an aria, if you have the talent
Light to moderate	You're working, but not too hard	• Breathing easily • Sweating lightly • Still finding it easy to talk or sing
Moderate	You're working	• Breathing faster • Starting to sweat more • Able to talk, not able to sing
Moderate to high	You're really working	• Huffing and puffing • Sweating • Able to talk in short sentences, but concentrating more on exercise than conversation
High	You're working very hard, almost out of gas	• Breathing hard • Sweating hard • Finding talking difficult

Exercise 101 | **SPECIAL SECTION**

strength workout on Tuesday, don't repeat it before Thursday.

3 Flexibility exercises

Flexibility exercises like stretching, yoga, and Pilates gently reverse the shortening and weakening of muscles that typically occur as you age. Shorter, stiffer muscle fibers may make you vulnerable to injuries and contribute to back pain and balance problems. Plus, secretions designed to lubricate muscles tend to dry up as you grow older.

The good news? Frequently performing exercises that isolate and stretch elastic fibers surrounding muscles and tendons helps counteract this decline. Encouraging blood flow to muscles makes them more limber. And a well-stretched muscle more easily achieves its full range of motion, which improves athletic performance. If you're a tennis player, you could reach an overhead you might have missed. Or think about a golfer who is able to swing with greater ease and less restriction. Likewise, reaching, bending, and stooping during daily tasks may be easier, and a hard-to-reach shoelace or fastener may now be within grasp.

At one time, experts prescribed stretching before exercise to help people sidestep injuries. Newer research suggests this does no good. It's better to stretch when your muscles are warm and pliable by folding flexibility exercises into your post-workout cool-down. Stretching between exercises may be fine, too, and possibly helps boost flexibility, as shown in a study on lower-leg and ankle stretching sponsored by the American College of Sports Medicine (ACSM).

How often to perform: The ACSM recommends doing flexibility exercises at least two to three times a week. Hold stretches for 10 to 30 seconds, repeating each stretch four times.

4 Balance exercises

Want to improve stability, which tends to erode as you age? Balance exercises can help you do just that. They offer an excellent defense against falls, which can be far more dangerous than you might imagine. Often, falls cause head injuries and temporarily or permanently disabling bone fractures. Balance typically worsens over time, compromised by medical conditions, medications, changes in vision, and lack of flexibility. Activities that enhance balance include tai chi, yoga, Pilates, and numerous exercises in this report designed to challenge stability.

How often to perform: Two to seven days a week.

5 Relaxation exercises

Relaxation exercises are not, strictly speaking, a component of most fitness programs. Yet stress reduction enhances quality of life and health. Some disciplines like Pilates, yoga, and tai chi meld tension-melting movements with mental focus and meditation. While improving strength, flexibility, and balance, practitioners ease stress, relieve pain, and gain an overall sense of well-being. Even walking can be a meditative practice (see "Treat your mind and body to a mindful walk," page 14). Stretching, too, releases muscle tension and promotes inner calm.

How often to perform: Incorporate a daily dose of relaxation.

Terms to know

What are power training, interval training, periodization, task-specific training, and complex workouts? They are five ways to juice up a workout, as described below.

Power training

Muscle power is the intersection of speed and strength: how quickly you can exert a given force to produce a desired movement. Strength in your leg muscles helps you walk across a four-lane intersection; speed moves you swiftly enough to beat the light. When not tuned up, speed ebbs even more quickly than muscle strength as you age. That means to maintain power over the years, it's important to focus on speed in at least some of your workouts. Power training may hinge on fast, explosive moves like the plyometric jumps in the "Power challenge workout" (see page 41), or require you to do exercises at your usual pace while wearing a weighted vest. Athletes often use power moves tailored to their sports in order to bump up their game.

Interval training

Interval training consists of bursts of vigorous activity alternating with lower-intensity activity. You might jump rope for a minute, then walk briskly for three minutes, then repeat the pattern. Or break up your usual walk by jogging—or sprinting—at regular intervals. Interval training alternates aerobic activities, which use oxygen to turn stored glycogen into energy, and anaerobic activities, which don't need oxygen to make the energy conversion. Training this way delivers cardiovascular benefits and challenges muscles sufficiently to strengthen them. Additionally, it can bump you up to the next level if your exercise reaches a plateau.

Periodization

Periodization is a training technique based on the idea that muscles adapt to challenges. A weight that's initially hard to lift becomes less challenging as your muscle grows stronger. If you keep using the same weight or doing exactly the same exercise routine, for example, your muscles stop improving.

Periodization helps you avoid overuse injuries and improve fitness by changing up your workout periodically—every five to six weeks is typical, but time frames vary from person to person. Switching to a new workout challenges different muscle groups and often builds different components of fitness.

An equally important reason is compliance. It's easy to get bored by an exercise routine. Creating variety makes exercise more interesting and fun. Fitness pros and athletes use periodization in very specific ways to train for sports events.

Task-specific training

Often, exercises are designed to isolate specific muscles—biceps, let's say, or knee extensors—to work on building them up. Task-specific training takes a different approach by working multiple muscle groups through dynamic movements similar to those you might make in sports or daily life. Depending on its focus, task-specific training can bolster athletic performance or basic abilities.

Many of the workouts in this report include this type of training. An exercise in which you swing your arm up while rotating at the waist (see "External arm rotation with diagonal reach," page 24) helps hone muscle sets you might use in golf, tennis, squash, or volleyball. Explosive jumps from one side of a rope to the other (see "Lateral jump," page 43) build muscles used in skiing, basketball, and soccer. Meanwhile, squats and chair stands strengthen muscles that allow you to sit, rise from a seat, and walk up stairs—all tasks important for independent living.

Complex workouts

These workouts braid together two or more exercises into a single sequence. Flowing from one exercise—and muscle group—to the next without pausing for a rest between each exercise delivers a strong, time-efficient workout. For example, one set might be eight to 12 reps of a sequence requiring a bridge, leg extension, and hamstring curl, followed by a rest before starting a second set. (For definitions of terms like "reps" and "sets," see "Key to the instructions," page 17.) Complex workouts are an excellent way to add variety to your exercise routine, often while increasing the challenge. ♥

Measuring gains

Tracking progress often helps keep you motivated. You can do that with old-fashioned paper and pencil or with one of the many apps available, such as My Fitness Pal or Nike Training Club. Exercise tools also abound online, at sites like these:

- **The President's Council** lets you create an account to track your progress as an individual or a family at www.presidentschallenge.org.
- **Exercise Prescription** includes over 1,400 exercises that can be tailored to your needs, along with fitness assessment calculators, at www.ExRx.net.
- **Map My Run** and **Map My Ride** help you create routes for running and biking and track your progress at www.mapmyrun.com and its counterpart, www.mapmyride.com.

Formal measures

Six weeks of workouts won't set you up for Muscle Beach, but you should start noticing gains at or before that point. If you want to find out whether your exercise routine is improving your cardiovascular fitness or making you more limber, keep a record of your workout times and results. There are number of valid measures you can use. Here are some of the more formal ways of measuring gains.

■ **Cardio.** Map out a course for walking, running, biking, or swimming laps in a pool. Time yourself initially to get your baseline. Every few weeks, repeat this test and note any improvements.

■ **Strength.** Do the concentrated biceps curl (page 40) and traveling side squats (page 25). Select a weight that tires the muscle by the last two reps in an eight-rep set. This is your baseline. In four to six weeks, repeat this test. Are you able to use a heavier weight or resistance band?

■ **Flexibility.** Do the hamstring stretch from our cool-down (page 47) or the sit-and-reach test described in the President's Challenge Adult Fitness Test (www.health.harvard.edu/sitreach). Every few weeks, repeat the exercise to see if you can comfortably stretch farther or hold the stretch longer.

■ **Balance.** For your baseline, time how long you can stand on each leg. Every few weeks, repeat the test.

Other measures

You can also try the following to take stock of the changes regular workouts make in your body and your health.

■ **Take your vitals.** Every few weeks, jot down your resting heart rate (before you rise in the morning) and blood pressure. Both tend to be lower in people who exercise regularly, so you may notice a healthy trend downward.

■ **Crack out the measuring tape.** Before you start a regular program of exercise, carefully measure your waist at its smallest circumference. If you like, also measure calves, upper thighs, and upper arms at their largest circumference. Make measurements again after six weeks. Over time, you may be gaining muscle mass in some spots (bigger biceps, perhaps) and toning up in others (smaller waist).

■ **Check your closet.** Perhaps you have a favorite pair of "skinny jeans" that can serve as your fitness barometer by loosening up or just skimming your body nicely when you work out regularly. Maybe you look sleeker (or more muscular) in a sleeveless shirt or bathing suit.

■ **Notice whether you feel fitter.** Are you huffing less when you take the stairs? Biking or hiking with increasing ease? Scooping up several heavy bags of groceries to make one trip inside, rather than two? Able to run or walk faster or for longer stretches of time? All of this counts toward health and quality of life. ♥

Gym versus home

No one needs to join a gym to exercise regularly. As many of the exercises we've selected for our workouts attest, your body offers the cheapest equipment available. A small investment in additional equipment—such as hand weights, resistance tubing, and a stability ball—greatly expands your exercise options.

Gyms do have advantages, though. Monthly fees are a big incentive to exercise. Classes offer companionship, a chance to learn proper technique, and opportunities to challenge your body and sample new trends (see "Try new trends," page 13). Gyms can afford sturdy equipment that would drain your bank account and overflow floor space at home. Often personal trainers are available for weekly appointments, small group training sessions, or a short-term overhaul to freshen your routine (see "Working with a personal trainer," below). Also, for many people being around others who are investing time and effort in their physical fitness is motivating.

When looking for a gym, consider these questions:
- Based on your goals, which amenities will you really use (classes, trainers, showers and sauna, or just gym equipment)? Watch out for additional amenities that hike up cost.
- How busy is the gym at the times you expect to work out? Is there sufficient equipment so you won't waste time waiting?
- Can you test-drive the gym with a free pass for a day or week?
- Is equipment in good shape and sized to fit you?
- Are staff members well-trained, pleasant, and appropriately certified and experienced?
- Is everything clean and well-maintained?
- Are there ways to trim membership costs to fit your pocketbook? You might save money by working out only during off-peak hours, selecting a gym with limited amenities, or choosing community centers, storefront gyms, or branches of the Y.

Working with a personal trainer

While you can certainly follow our workouts on your own, personal trainers have valuable skills for you to tap. Among the things they can do for you, they can
- motivate and cheer you on
- safely push you to the next level
- teach you new skills while fine-tuning your form
- tailor an exercise program to any goals you choose: enhancing health and appearance, losing weight, charging through a triathlon, or another aim entirely
- keep boredom at bay by changing up routines.

Choosing a trainer

No nationwide licensing requirements exist for personal trainers. So in addition to seeking a good match in personalities and respect for your goals, you should ask about these points:

Certification. Two well-respected certifying organizations are the American College of Sports Medicine (ACSM) and American Council on Exercise (ACE); others include the National Council on Strength and Fitness (NCSF), National Strength and Conditioning Association (NSCA), and National Academy of Sports Medicine (NASM), or other groups whose certifications are recognized by the National Commission for Certifying Agencies (NCCA).

Experience. Years of experience matter, as does experience in working with others like you, whether you're a gifted athlete or a confirmed sloth with tricky knees. Some trainers specialize in working with particular populations—older adults, athletes—and may have taken courses and possibly certifying exams in these areas.

References. Personal recommendations from friends count in choosing a trainer. Local gyms may list their trainers, and certifying organizations like ACE and ACSM often have referral systems. Try to call a few references.

Liability insurance. Gyms may have liability insurance that covers their trainers, but it's best to ask. Ask independent trainers that question, too.

Try new trends

Kickboxing and rebounding. Zumba, spinning, and Indo-Row. Boot camp and belly dancing. Pilates begat Yogalates, and the once ubiquitous hatha yoga now supports an apparently endless stream of variations.

Exercisers have restless souls, it seems, and new group workouts and equipment constantly crop up to feed the demand. Sampling new classes at your gym or at studios run by independent trainers is an enjoyable way to re-energize dull exercise routines. Ask whether a range of beginner to advanced classes is available to bring you up to speed on a new routine or jump you to a higher level. The guide below is an introduction to just a few of the trends.

■ **Barre classes** are all the rage now at several boutique studio chains and many gyms. Exercises are performed at a ballet barre and focus on individual muscle groups, alignment, flexibility, and posture. They do not include a large aerobic component, but the work on individual muscles can be intense.

■ **Belly dancing** is a refreshing way to isolate and work abdominal muscles to rhythms that inspire sensual, flexible movements.

■ **Boot camps** have spread like wildfire, each one boasting its own brand of cardio and strength moves designed to prod muscle growth and fitness improvements in those dedicated enough to slog through arduous workouts several times a week. Some boot camp instructors seem to be channeling old Army training videos ("Drop and give me 50!"). Others mix martial arts moves or hefty weights like kettle bells into the routine.

■ **CrossFit** is a regimen of high-intensity interval training that is included in some boot camps. Although beneficial to some, it should be undertaken slowly and within one's own limits.

■ **Indo-Row** is a full-body workout on rowing machines that combines cardio and strength with an emphasis on core training. Background music pumps away while an instructor guides the class through intervals of rowing sprints and slower drills.

■ **Kickboxing,** one of many martial art variations, offers a high-energy cardio workout that enhances balance as you punch, kick, and lunge.

■ **Pilates,** like yoga, is an umbrella term covering many teaching styles. Over all, Pilates enhances flexibility, core strength, balance, and relaxation. Controlled breathing, correct postural alignment, and positive visualization are central to all forms of it. An emphasis on small, flowing moves and a long, lean silhouette appeals to dancers, gymnasts, and many non-athletes, particularly people looking for low-impact activities. Pilates equipment includes weighted hand balls, resistance bands or straps, and a padded apparatus called the Reformer that employs a flat, sliding platform plus pulleys, cables, and straps for resistance.

■ **Plyometrics,** or jump training, is a powerful, explosive endurance workout that employs movements familiar from sports like skiing, basketball, and tennis. Muscles are stretched before a jump, quickly contract during the jump, then are stretched again on the landing. (This is not the workout to choose if you're in poor condition or have orthopedic problems that jumping may exacerbate.)

■ **Rebounding** kicks cardio up a notch by having you perform familiar aerobic moves and jumps on a small trampoline. It's easy on the joints and superb for stability.

■ **Spinning** is a group cardio workout on bikes that slides from pedaling at slow speeds to mashing down at rates reminiscent of the Tour de France that send heartbeats into the stratosphere. Thumping music helps set the pace.

■ **Tabata** is a type of high-intensity interval training that is often taught at gyms.

■ **Yoga** once came in only a single flavor—marked by iconic, meditative poses and deep, calming breaths—for all but the most enlightened. That's not

Treat your mind and body to a mindful walk

Mindfulness is a technique that encourages you to slow a racing mind and embrace each moment as it unfolds. Blended with a simple, repetitive exercise like walking, running, or swimming, it is a wonderful way to ease stress. By fully engaging all of your senses, mindfulness teaches you to focus attention on what is happening in the present and accept it without judgment. This enhances your appreciation of simple everyday experiences, such as the walk described below.

A mindful walk

As you walk, first narrow your concentration by focusing on an aspect of your breathing: the sensations of air flowing into your nostrils and out of your mouth, your belly expanding as you inhale and contracting as you exhale. Try counting from one to five as you inhale, then five to one as you exhale. Do this for a few minutes. Then begin to widen your focus. While you continue breathing in and out in a measured way, open up your senses to become aware of sounds, scents, and sensations. Enjoy the rhythmic thump of each foot hitting the ground and the whisper of clothes rubbing lightly against each other. Feel the touch of a cool or warm breeze against your face, notice light and shadows cast on you as you move, or soak in the sun beaming down. Listen for natural sounds even when walking on city blocks: the chirp of crickets or hum of cicadas, bird songs, rustling leaves, wind blowing. As you tune in to your breathing, your body, and your surroundings, you will notice much beyond these examples. Throughout your walk, continue to breathe slowly and deeply while remaining fully aware and staying in the moment.

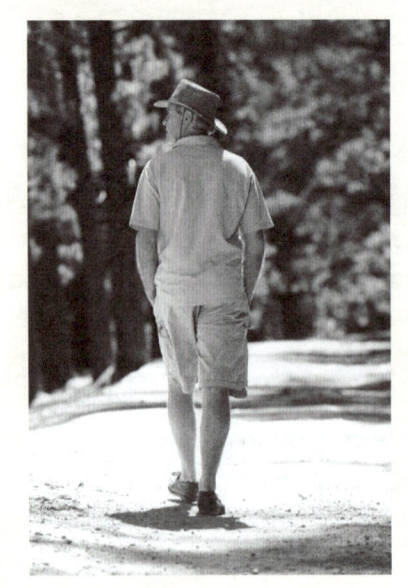

Try not to rush. Proceed slowly and with deliberation, engaging your senses fully to savor every sensation. If your mind starts to race, return your focus to your breathing. Then expand your awareness again. Consider how you feel physically and psychologically before, during, and after your walk.

---

the case anymore. Generally, different styles of yoga offer a mix of flexibility, balance, and relaxation activities, sometimes with strengthening moves folded in. Hatha yoga refers to a basic, gentle class that can serve as a wonderful introduction to the classic poses and meditation. Power yoga pushes muscles to the brink with advanced poses held for long periods. Bikram yoga takes practitioners through well over 20 poses in a hotter-than-body-heat room, a touch that loosens muscles and opens pores. Ashtanga yoga is another demanding workout using a set group of poses with many athletic flourishes, such as back bends and handstands. Iyengar yoga focuses on striking perfect positions during poses, sometimes using props like straps or blocks to assist. Vinyasa yoga centers on breathing and a smooth flow from pose to pose. Kundalini yoga releases energy through chanting and a series of poses carefully combined with measured breathing.

- **Yogilates** and **Yogalates,** two popular offshoots created separately by two trainers, marry the core work done in Pilates with the flexibility, strength, and spirituality emphasized in yoga.

- **Zumba** encourages flexibility and pours on the cardio through sensual dance moves like salsa, meringue, and cumbia set to infectious Latin and international beats. Zumba has its own spin-offs: Zumba Gold is for people 60 and older; Zumba Toning employs weighted sticks to sculpt and tone.

Avoiding injury

Before starting a new exercise program, should you talk to a doctor about whether you need to start slowly or take any precautions, like avoiding certain exercises? Almost anybody can safely take up walking, and light-to-moderate exercise is usually fine for healthy adults with no troublesome symptoms. But it's wise to talk to a doctor if you have any questions about your health or plan to start strenuous workouts, especially if you haven't been active recently.

One helpful resource for gauging your ability is the Canadian Society for Exercise Physiologists' updated Physical Activity Readiness Questionnaire (PAR-Q+; www.health.harvard.edu/par-q). Definitely talk to a doctor if you have any injuries or a chronic or unstable health condition, such as heart disease, asthma, high blood pressure, osteoporosis, or diabetes.

In some cases, your doctor may suggest you meet with a physiatrist. Physiatrists are physicians who specialize in rehabilitation. They focus on treating—and helping to prevent—nerve, muscle, and bone conditions that affect how you move. Back problems, knee or shoulder injuries, debilitating arthritis or obesity, stroke, and repetitive stress injuries are a few examples of these conditions. A physiatrist can tailor an exercise prescription to enhance recovery after surgery or injury, or to work with the limitations posed by chronic problems that interfere with exercise by sparking pain or limiting movements. He or she can also tell you whether certain types of exercises will be helpful or harmful given your situation.

Safety first

Once you have the go-ahead to exercise, follow these guidelines to ensure a safe workout:

- Take time to warm up and cool down properly (see "Warm-up," page 19, and "Cool-down," page 47).
- Never sacrifice good form and posture for the sake of lifting heavier weights or finishing a set (see "Posture and alignment: Striking the right pose," page 16).
- Boost your activity level gradually. Unless you already exercise frequently and vigorously, plan to work your way up to the "Complex challenge workout" (page 44) rather than starting with it.
- Don't train too hard or too often. Either can cause overuse injuries like stress fractures, stiff or sore joints and muscles, and inflamed tendons and ligaments. Sports prompting repetitive wear and tear on certain parts of your body—such as swimming (shoulders), jogging (knees, ankles, and feet), and tennis (elbows)—are often overuse culprits, too. A mix of workouts, sports, and rest is safer.
- Pay attention to your body. Don't exercise when you're sick or fatigued from overtraining. Fatigue may increase your risk of injuries. Note that your joints should never hurt as a result of exercise. If they do, stop the exercise you're doing.
- If you go for weeks or months without exercising, drop back if necessary when you start again by lifting lighter weights, choosing an easier workout, or doing fewer reps or sets.
- Stay hydrated while exercising, especially when it's hot or humid. If you're working out especially hard or doing a marathon or triathlon, choose drinks that replace fluids plus essential electrolytes.
- Choose clothes and shoes designed for your type of exercise. Replace shoes every six months as cushioning wears out.
- Pay attention to muscle soreness. Soreness that begins 12 to 24 hours after exercise is normal. But if you have persistent or intense muscle pain that starts during a workout or right afterward, or persists more than one to two weeks, call your doctor.
- In hot, humid weather, watch for signs of overheating, such as headache, dizziness, nausea, faintness, cramps, or palpitations. And make it a point to exercise during cooler morning or evening hours or at an air-conditioned gym.

- Any time you exercise, it's safest to call your doctor for advice if you experience notable dizziness or faintness, chest pain, or significant or persistent shortness of breath.

Posture and alignment: Striking the right pose

Exercise is important, but if you don't do it right, you run the risk of injuring yourself. Working to achieve good form means more gains and fewer injuries.

Posture helps more than you might think. In fact, good posture and alignment help anytime you're moving. If one foot is always turned slightly inward, for example, it impedes power whether you're walking, going upstairs, jogging, or playing sports. The exercises in our workouts often call for you to stand up straight. That means

- your chin is parallel to the floor
- both shoulders are even (roll them up, back, and down to help achieve this)
- both wrists are firm and straight, not flexed upward or downward
- both hips are even
- both knees are even and pointed straight ahead
- both feet are pointed straight ahead
- body weight is distributed evenly on both feet.

In addition, it's important to maintain a neutral spine. A neutral spine takes into account the slight natural curves of the spine, but it's not flexed or arched. One way to find the neutral position is to tip your pelvis forward as far as comfortable, then tip it backward as far as is comfortable. The spot approximately in the middle should be neutral. If you're not used to standing or sitting up straight, it may take a while for this to feel natural.

Few of us have perfect posture, which is why it's so important to check your posture before and during each exercise. Looking in a mirror as you do exercises helps enormously.

6 tips for effective strength training

1. Focus on form, not weight. In addition to causing injuries, poor form can slow gains because you aren't isolating muscles properly. Start off with very light weights in order to get your alignment and form right. Concentrate on performing slow, smooth lifts and equally controlled descents while isolating a muscle group. You isolate a muscle group by holding your body in a specific position while consciously contracting and releasing those muscles.

2. Tempo, tempo. Control is very important. Tempo helps you stay in control rather than undercut gains through momentum. Sometimes switching speed—for example, lowering for three counts, lifting for one count—is a useful technique for enhancing power. Follow the tempo specified in each exercise for better gains.

3. Breathe. Blood pressure rises if you hold your breath while performing strength exercises. Exhale as you work against gravity by lifting, pushing, or pulling; inhale as you release.

4. Keep challenging muscles. For best results, choose a weight that tires the targeted muscle or muscles by the last two reps while still allowing you to maintain good form. If you can't do the last two reps, choose a lighter weight. As you grow stronger, challenge your muscles again by adding weight (roughly 1 to 2 pounds for arms, 2 to 5 pounds for legs); adding a set to your workout (up to three sets); or working out additional days per week (as long as you rest muscle groups 48 hours between strength workouts).

5. Practice regularly. Performing a complete upper- and lower-body strength workout two or three times a week is ideal.

6. Give muscles time off. Strenuous exercise like strength training causes tiny tears in muscle tissue. Muscles grow stronger as the tears knit up. Always allow at least 48 hours between sessions for muscles to recover. If you do split strength sessions, you might do upper body on Monday, lower body on Tuesday, upper body on Wednesday, lower body on Thursday, etc.

The workouts

From warm-up to cool-down and everything in between, our nine workouts offer you the benefits of strength training, as well as flexibility, balance, and relaxation exercises. Table 2 (below) sketches out the multiple benefits you can derive from each routine.

Note, however, that while these workouts focus a great deal on strength training, they include less aerobic exercise, since people generally have an easier time figuring out how to get this type of exercise—with a brisk walk, for example, or 30 minutes on the elliptical machine at the gym. Whatever option you choose, the Physical Activity Guidelines for Americans call for 150 minutes of moderate-intensity aerobic activity per week, in addition to two strength-training sessions, so definitely augment the workouts here with aerobic training. (For ideas, see "Try new trends," page 13.)

Key to the instructions

Each of the exercises in our workouts includes certain directions. We describe your starting position and the movement you will make, along with tips and techniques to help. We also use certain terms you'll need to know.

- **Repetitions (or reps).** Each time you perform the movement in an exercise, that's called a rep. If you cannot do all the reps at first, just do what you can, and then gradually increase reps as you improve.
- **Set.** One set is a specific number of repetitions. For example, 10 to 12 reps often make a single set. Usually, we suggest doing one to three sets.
- **Supersets.** These are paired exercises. Normally, you perform a set, then rest and repeat the set. During a superset, you perform all the reps of exercise A, then immediately move on to do all the reps of exercise

Table 2: Fitness gains from Harvard workouts

Many new exercise routines—including the nine great workouts our personal trainers designed for you (see pages 19–48)—fulfill several fitness goals at once by combining aerobic and strength benefits, for example, or strength, flexibility, and relaxation.

WORKOUT	CARDIO	STRENGTH	FLEXIBILITY	BALANCE	RELAXATION
Warm-up* (page 19)	★		★		
Home and travel workout (page 20)		★		★	
Resistance band and tube workout (page 23)		★		★	
Ball workout (page 26)		★	★	★	
Mixed workout: Bosu, weights, and medicine ball (page 29)	★	★		★	
Core workout (page 32)		★		★	
Split strength workout: Lower body (page 35)		★		★	
Split strength workout: Upper body (page 38)		★			
Power challenge workout (page 41)	★	★		★	
Complex challenge workout (page 44)		★		★	
Cool-down (page 47)			★	★	★

* While the warm-up is largely cardio, it's typically too short to count toward health goals.

B. Then you rest and repeat the entire superset. Supersets make a workout more vigorous. Boxes on some workouts note which exercises pair well as supersets so you can choose to do the exercise routine as written or juice it up with a superset. Our "Complex challenge workout" (page 44) also relies on supersets.

■ **Intensity.** Intensity measures how hard you work during an exercise. Pay attention to cues like breathing, talking, and sweating, or measure intensity through perceived exertion (see Table 1, page 8).

■ **Tempo.** This tells you the count for the key movements in an exercise. For example, 1-3 means lift a weight in one count, then lower it on a count of three. Two other examples are 4-4 (lift in four counts, no pause at all, lower in four counts) and 2-2-2-2 (lift in two counts, rotate right in two counts, rotate back to center in two counts, lower in two counts). Here's how the 2-1-2 tempo works during the movements in the wall push-up: Slowly count to two while bending your elbows to lower your upper body toward the wall. Pause for one count. Then take two counts to return to the starting position.

■ **Hold.** Hold tells you the number of seconds to pause while holding a pose during an exercise. You'll see this in stretches, which are held for up to 30 seconds, and for the plank exercises.

■ **Rest.** Resting gives your muscles a chance to recharge and helps you maintain good form. Except during the warm-up and cool-down activities, we specify a range of time to rest between sets (and sometimes between reps, for especially tiring exercises). How much of this time you need will differ depending on your level of fitness, how heavy your weights are if you are strength training, and the intensity of the exercises.

Equipment used in the workouts

Our "Home and travel workout" (page 20) requires no special gear. But the other workouts that follow do call for some basic equipment, which you can either buy or use at the gym.

■ **Ankle weights** (for strength exercises). Look for comfortably padded ankle cuffs with pockets designed to hold half-pound or pound weight bars to add as you progress. Ankle weight sets are usually 5 to 10 pounds. A single cuff may suffice, depending on the exercises you intend to do.

■ **Body Bar** (for strength exercises). This padded bar comes in various weights, starting with 3 or 6 pounds.

■ **Bosu** (for core and balance exercises). A Bosu essentially is half a stability ball (see below) mounted on a heavy rubber platform that helps hold it firmly in place. Though it can be used with either side up—the ball or the rubber platform—all our exercises call for the ball side to face up. In this position, fully inflating the Bosu to nine inches in height makes it firmer and more stable; inflating it less increases instability, which is helpful for more advanced balance and core work.

■ **Exercise mat** (for floor exercises). Choose a non-slip, well-padded mat. A thick carpet or towels will do in a pinch.

■ **Hand weights** (for strength exercises). Depending on your current strength, start with sets of weights as low as 2 pounds and 5 pounds or 5 pounds and 8 pounds. Add heavier weights as needed. Dumbbells with padded center bars and D-shaped weights are easy to hold. Kits that let you screw weights onto a central bar are available, too.

■ **Medicine balls** (for core and strength exercises). The balls come in different weights and are similar in size to a soccer ball or basketball. Some have a handle on top. A 4- to 6-pound medicine ball is a good start for most people.

■ **Resistance bands** (for strength exercises). These look like big, wide rubber bands and come in several levels of resistance, designated by color.

■ **Resistance tubing** (for strength exercises). Look for tubing with padded handles on each end in several levels of resistance. Different colors designate varying amounts of resistance from very light to very heavy. Some brands come with a door attachment helpful for anchoring the tubing in place when doing certain exercises.

■ **Stability ball** (for core work, stretching, and balance exercises). Stability balls come in several sizes (55 cm, 65 cm, 75 cm are most common, but smaller and larger balls are available). Check the size chart linked to height to select a ball. When you sit on a ball, your hips and knees should both be at a 90-degree angle. Be sure to buy a durable, high-grade ball. ♥

Warm-up

Warming up pumps nutrient-rich, oxygenated blood to your muscles as it speeds up your heart rate and breathing. A good warm-up should last five to 10 minutes and work all major muscle groups. Start slowly, then pick up the pace. Usually, you would rest between sets, but that's not necessary here. Instead, do one set of each exercise, then repeat from the top. If you prefer, you can do a simpler warm-up by walking in place while gently swinging your arms or dancing to a few songs.

Equipment: No equipment needed

1 | Alternating reach

Reps: 16 overhead and 16 across
Sets: 1–2
Intensity: Light to moderate
Tempo: 2-2
Rest: No rest needed

Starting position: Stand up straight with your feet hip-width apart and your hands at your sides.

Movement: Reach your right hand overhead, then bring it back down to your side. Repeat with your left hand. Finish all overhead reps, then return to the starting position and begin alternating reaches across your body at shoulder level toward the opposite front corners of the room. This is one complete set.

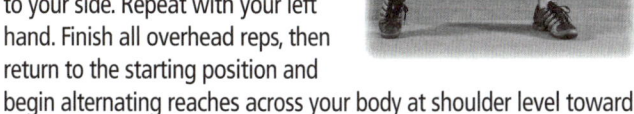

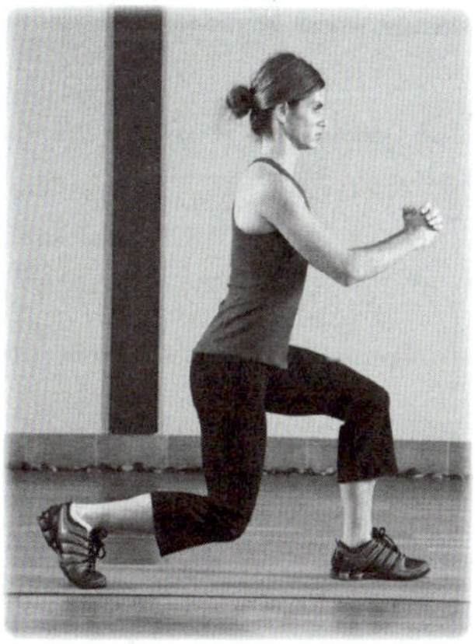

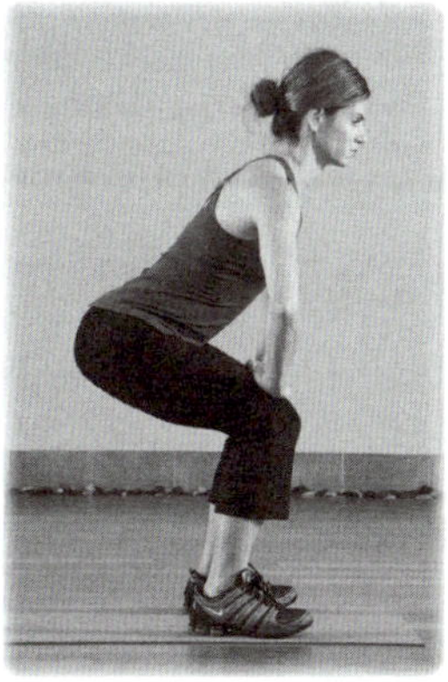

Tips and techniques:
- Keep moves rhythmic and controlled.
- Rotate your torso slightly when reaching across your body.

3 | Squat

Reps: 16
Sets: 1–2
Intensity: Moderate
Tempo: 2-2
Rest: No rest needed

Starting position: Stand up straight with your feet shoulder-width apart.

Movement: Hinge forward at your hips and bend your knees to lower your buttocks toward the floor as if sitting down in a chair, while resting your hands on your thighs. Stop with your buttocks above knee level. Return to the starting position.

Tips and techniques:
- Press your weight back into your heels when squatting.
- Don't extend your knees beyond the tips of your toes.
- Keep your spine neutral.

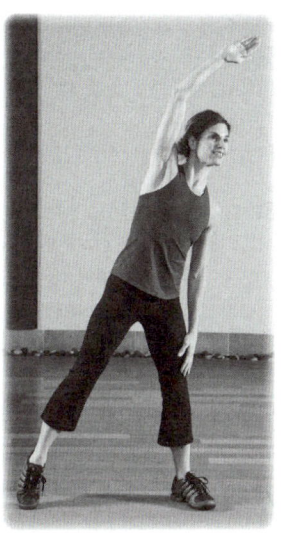

2 | Alternating knee lift

Reps: 16
Sets: 1–2
Intensity: Light to moderate
Tempo: 1-1
Rest: No rest needed

Starting position: Stand up straight with your feet together and your hands at your sides.

Movement: Lift your right knee toward the ceiling. Lower to the starting position. Repeat with your left knee.

Tips and techniques:
- Maintain upright posture throughout the move.
- Lift and lower your legs in a controlled manner.

4 | Reverse lunge

Reps: 16
Sets: 1–2
Intensity: Moderate
Tempo: 2-2
Rest: No rest needed

Starting position: Stand up straight with your feet together and your hands at your sides.

Movement: Step back on the ball of your right foot and sink into a lunge, clasping your hands loosely in front of your chest. Your left knee should align over your left ankle, and your right knee should point to the floor. Return to the starting position and step back on the ball of your left foot to do the lunge on the other side.

Tips and techniques:
- Keep your spine neutral when sinking into the lunge.
- As you bend your knees, lower the back knee directly down to the floor with the thigh perpendicular to the floor.

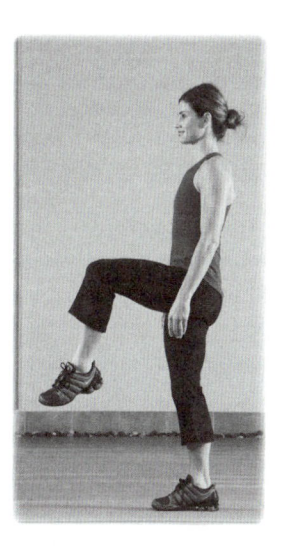

www.health.harvard.edu • Workout Workbook • 19

Home and travel workout

This full-body workout for home or travel requires practically no equipment. A sturdy chair and a comfortable spot for floor exercises is all you need. That leaves plenty of room in your closets—or carry-on bag—for clothes. Remember to bracket your workout with a warm-up and cool-down.

Equipment:
- Sturdy chair
- Mat, towels, or carpet for comfort during floor exercises

1 | Wall push-up

Reps: 8–12
Sets: 1–3
Intensity: Moderate
Tempo: 2-1-2
Rest: 30–90 seconds between sets

Starting position: Stand up straight in front of a wall with your arms extended at shoulder height. Put your palms against the wall with the fingers pointing upward.

Movement: Bend your elbows to lower your upper body as much as possible toward the wall, keeping a straight line from head to heel. Pause, then push away from the wall to return to the starting position, maintaining neutral alignment from head to toe throughout the movement.

Tips and techniques:
- Keep your hands no higher than shoulder level.
- Keep your elbows close to your sides as you bend them.
- Keep your shoulders down and back.

Too hard? Lower your upper body less toward the wall.
Too easy? Lift one foot a few inches off the floor behind you as you do the push-ups. Keep your arms at shoulder height and maintain neutral alignment.

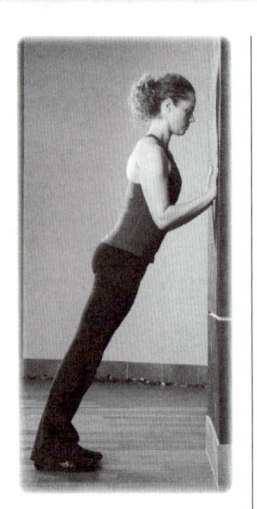

2 | Triceps dip

Reps: 8–12
Sets: 1–3
Intensity: Moderate to high
Tempo: 2-2
Rest: 30–90 seconds between sets

Starting position: Sit near the edge of a sturdy chair with your legs partly extended, knees bent, and heels touching the floor. Put your palms down on the chair next to your hips and curve your fingers over the edge. Pushing down on your hands, raise your buttocks up a bit and move them forward to clear the edge of the chair.

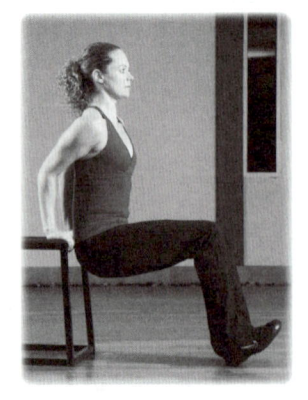

Movement: Bend your elbows and lower your hips toward the floor. Straighten your arms to return to the starting position.

Tips and techniques:
- Maintain a neutral spine throughout, keeping your back close to the chair.
- Keep your arms near your sides and your elbows pointing toward the back of the chair.
- Exhale as you extend your arms.

Too hard? Lower your body less toward the floor.
Too easy? Fully extend your legs in the starting position.

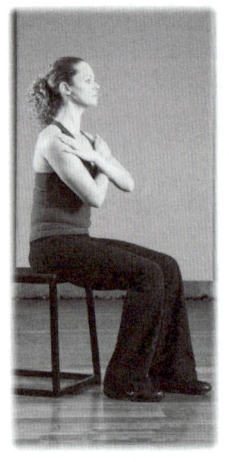

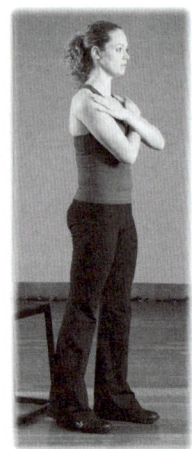

3 | Chair stand with staggered legs

Reps: 8–12 **Sets:** 1–3
Intensity: Moderate
Tempo: 3-1-3
Rest: 30–90 seconds between sets

Starting position: Sit up straight near the front edge of a sturdy chair with your arms crossed and fingers touching opposite shoulders. Position your feet hip-width apart and stagger them by moving one foot forward.

Movement: Smoothly stand up with your knees and hips pointing straight ahead. Pause, then return to the starting position.

After completing the 8–12 reps in one set, move the opposite foot forward and repeat the movement for the next set.

Tips and techniques:
- Maintain neutral posture throughout the movement.
- Tighten the muscles in your abdomen and buttocks.

Too hard? Line up your feet evenly, hip-width apart, in the starting position.
Too easy? Lift your arms over your head. Keep your shoulders down and back throughout the move.

Home and travel workout

4 | Bridge with chair

Reps: 8–12
Sets: 1–3
Intensity: Moderate
Tempo: 2-1-2
Rest: 30–90 seconds between sets

Starting position: Lie on your back with your knees bent and your arms at your sides, palms up. Put your heels on the seat of a chair placed so that your knees form a 90-degree angle. Relax your shoulders down and back into the floor.

Movement: Squeeze your buttocks as you lift your hips off the floor. Pause, then slowly release to return to the starting position.

Tips and techniques:
- Maintain a neutral spine throughout.
- Keep your shoulders, hips, and knees in a straight line during the bridge.

Too hard? Put both feet flat on the floor rather than on the chair.
Too easy? Put your left heel on the chair and extend your right leg toward the ceiling before doing the bridge. After completing the reps in one set, switch leg positions and repeat the movement for the next set.

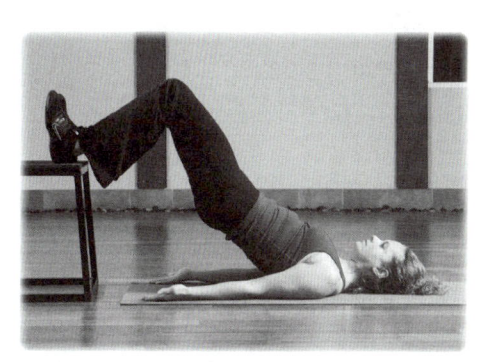

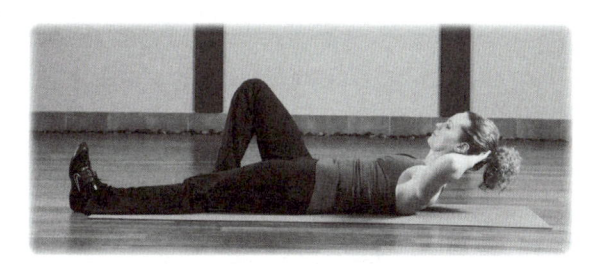

5 | Curl-up with one leg extended

Reps: 8–12
Sets: 1–3
Intensity: Moderate
Tempo: 2-1-2
Rest: 30–90 seconds between sets

Starting position: Lie on your back with your fingertips lightly behind your head, elbows out. Bend your right knee and place that foot flat on the floor while keeping your left leg extended.

Movement: Tighten your abdominal muscles. Lift your head and shoulders off the floor as you curl upward. Exhale as you lift. Pause, then return to the starting position.

Tips and techniques:
- Keep your fingertips resting lightly behind your head throughout the movement.
- If you have trouble maintaining a neutral neck, make a fist with one hand and place it under your chin for support.

Too hard? Put your fingertips behind your waist on the floor before starting the curl-up.
Too easy? Cross your arms over your chest before starting the curl-up, or increase the number of reps.

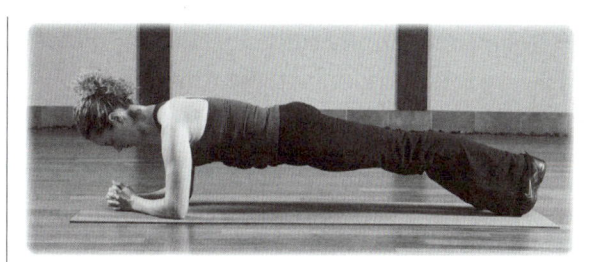

6 | Front plank

Reps: 2–4
Sets: 1
Intensity: Moderate to high
Hold: 15–60 seconds
Rest: 30–90 seconds between reps

Starting position: Start on your hands and knees.

Movement: Tighten your abdominal muscles and lower your upper body so that your forearms are on the floor, clasping your hands together and aligning your shoulders directly over your elbows. Extend both legs with your feet flexed and toes touching the floor so that you balance your body in a line like a plank. Hold. Breathe comfortably.

Tips and techniques:
- Keep your neck and spine in neutral alignment during the plank, not curving upward or downward.
- Keep your shoulders down and back.

Too hard? Put your knees on the floor instead of extending your legs.
Too easy? While holding your body in a line like a plank, lift your right foot and move it to the side six inches, tap the floor, and move it back to the center. Lift your left foot and move it to the side six inches, tap the floor, and move it back to the center. Continue for 15 to 60 seconds.

www.health.harvard.edu   Workout Workbook

Home and travel workout

7 | Standing side leg lift

Reps: 8–12 on each side
Sets: 1–3
Intensity: Moderate
Tempo: 2-1-2
Rest: 30–90 seconds between sets

Starting position: Stand up straight with your feet together and your hands on your hips.

Movement: Slowly lift your right leg straight out to the side. Pause, then slowly lower the leg. Keep your hips even throughout. Finish all reps before repeating with the leg positions reversed. This is one complete set.

Tips and techniques:
- Maintain neutral posture throughout.
- Tighten your abdominal muscles and squeeze the buttocks of the supporting leg.
- Exhale as you lift.

Too hard? Hold on to the back of a chair for balance and lift your leg a shorter distance.

Too easy? Hold for 4 counts at the top of the lift during each repetition.

8 | Heel raise

Reps: 8–12
Sets: 1–3
Intensity: Light to moderate
Tempo: 2-1-2
Rest: 30–90 seconds between sets

Starting position: Stand up straight with your hands on your hips.

Movement: Slowly rise up on the balls of both feet. Pause, then slowly lower your heels back to the floor.

Tips and techniques:
- Maintain neutral posture and tighten your buttock muscles for balance.
- As you lift, keep your ankles firm to avoid rolling to the outside of your foot.

Too hard? Hold on to the back of a chair for balance while doing the exercise.

Too easy? Try the exercise standing on your right leg only while lifting your left foot slightly off the floor. Finish all reps before repeating with the leg positions reversed. This is one complete set.

SUPERSET ME

Want to try supersets? Combine these:
- Bridge with chair + Curl-up with one leg extended
- Standing side leg lift + Heel raise

See "Supersets," page 17, for more information.

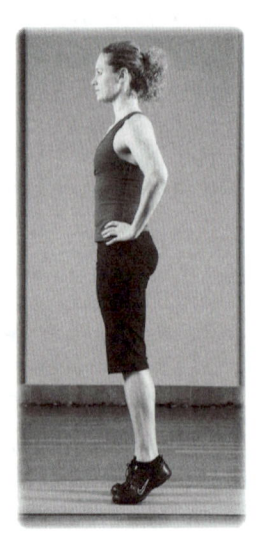

Resistance band and tube workout

Wide elastic resistance bands or resistance tubing with padded handles help build strength in this versatile, full-body workout. Bands and tubing come in varying levels of resistance indicated by different colors: depending on the brand, light resistance might be yellow, while medium resistance is orange, for example. Before doing most of these exercises, you must firmly anchor resistance tubing to a door or other structure. Some brands include a door attachment; if yours does not, you can wrap tubing around a column at the gym or around the leg of a heavy table or strong banister at home. Remember to bracket your workout with a warm-up and cool-down.

Equipment:
- Resistance bands
- Resistance tubing
- Stability ball

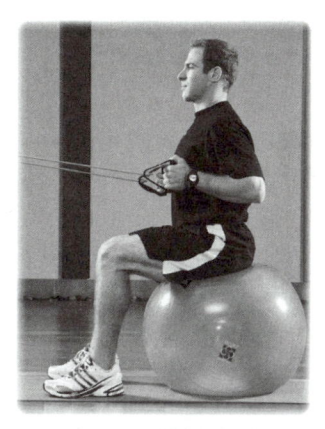

1 | Seated row on stability ball

Reps: 8–12
Sets: 1–3
Intensity: Moderate
Tempo: 4-4
Rest: 30–90 seconds between sets

Starting position: Anchor the resistance tubing so that it will be at chest height when you sit on a stability ball. Sit on the stability ball with your feet hip-width apart and hold the handles of the resistance tubing with your arms extended.

Movement: Squeeze your shoulder blades together. Slowly bend your arms and pull back, keeping your elbows close to your ribs and pointing toward the back wall. Slowly return to the starting position.

Tips and techniques:
- Keep your spine neutral and shoulders down and back.
- Keep your wrists firm.
- Keep the movement slow and controlled throughout.

Too hard? Sit on a chair instead of a stability ball. Use lighter resistance tubing.
Too easy? Use heavier resistance tubing.

SUPERSET ME

Want to try supersets? Combine these:
- Lat pull-down on stability ball + Chest press
- Squat + Traveling side squat

See "Supersets," page 17, for more information.

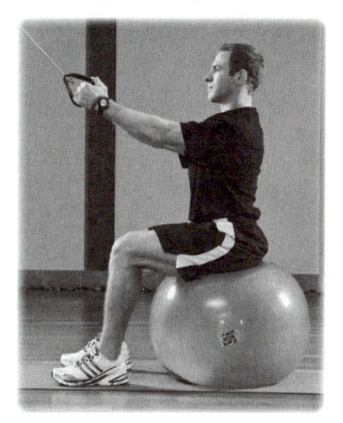

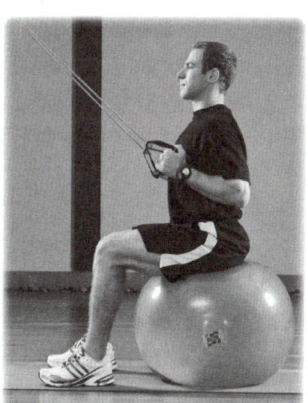

2 | Lat pull-down on stability ball

Reps: 8–12
Sets: 1–3
Intensity: Moderate
Tempo: 4-4
Rest: 30–90 seconds between sets

Starting position: Anchor the resistance tubing to the top of a door. Sit on a stability ball (facing the door) with your feet hip-width apart and hold on to the handles of the resistance tubing with your arms fully extended as if reaching toward the anchor point.

Movement: Slowly pull the handles of the resistance tubing back and down toward your ribs. Slowly return to the starting position.

Tips and techniques:
- Squeeze your shoulder blades together throughout the movement.
- Maintain upright posture throughout the exercise.
- Keep your shoulders down and back.

Too hard? Use lighter resistance tubing.
Too easy? Use heavier resistance tubing.

www.health.harvard.edu   Workout Workbook

Resistance band and tube workout

3 | Chest press

Reps: 8–12
Sets: 1–3
Intensity: Moderate
Tempo: 2-2
Rest: 30–90 seconds between sets

Starting position: Anchor the resistance tubing at chest level. Stand with your feet staggered and your back to the anchor point. Hold the handles of the tubing with your hands at your shoulders and elbows bent, pointing out to the side at a height even with your hands.

Movement: Fully extend both arms as you press forward at chest level, then return to the starting position.

Tips and techniques:
- Maintain neutral posture, keeping your shoulders down and back.
- Keep your movements slow, and control the tension on the tube throughout the exercise.
- Exhale as you press forward.

Too hard? Use lighter resistance tubing.
Too easy? Use heavier resistance tubing.

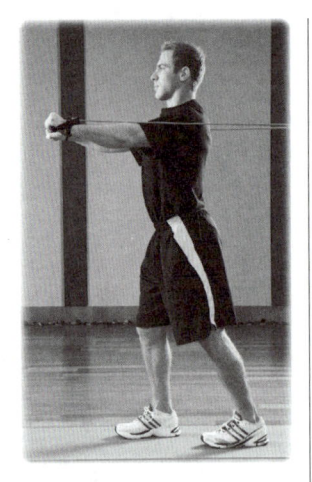

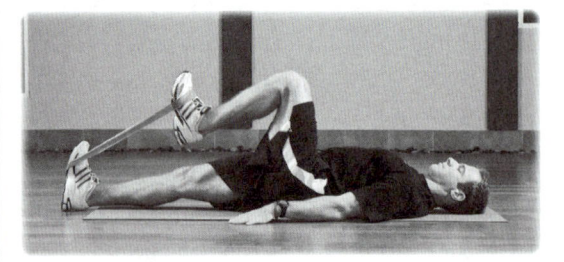

4 | Hip flexion

Reps: 8–12 on each side
Sets: 1–3
Intensity: Moderate to high
Tempo: 2-2
Rest: 30–90 seconds between sets

Starting position: Place a resistance band around your feet. Lie on your back with your hands at your sides and legs extended, heels on the floor.

Movement: Lift your right leg a few inches off the floor and pull your right knee in toward your chest. Pause, then extend your leg to return to the starting position. Finish all reps before repeating with the leg positions reversed. This is one complete set.

Tips and techniques:
- Keep your movements slow, and control the tension on the band throughout the exercise.
- Exhale as you pull your knee toward your chest.
- Maintain a neutral spine.

Too hard? Don't pull your knee in as close to your chest.
Too easy? Pull your knee in closer toward your chest.

5 | External arm rotation with diagonal reach

Reps: 8–12 on each side
Sets: 1–3
Intensity: Moderate
Tempo: 3-1-3
Rest: 30–90 seconds between sets

Starting position: Stand with your legs hip-width apart, chest up, and shoulders down and back. Anchor the middle of the resistance tubing to the floor with your left foot. Hold the handle of the resistance tubing in your right hand with your wrist straight and your hand near your left hip.

Movement: Keeping your wrist firm, lift up your right hand on a diagonal as if raising a racquet. Pause, then slowly return to the starting position. Finish all reps with right arm before anchoring the resistance tubing under your right foot and repeating with the left arm. This is one complete set.

Tips and techniques:
- Adjust the resistance tubing as needed so that you are able to do the movement with a full range of motion. Moving your foot closer to the handle in your hand increases resistance; moving your foot farther away from that handle decreases resistance.
- Keep your wrist firm and shoulders down and back throughout the movement.
- Keep your knees and hips pointing forward.

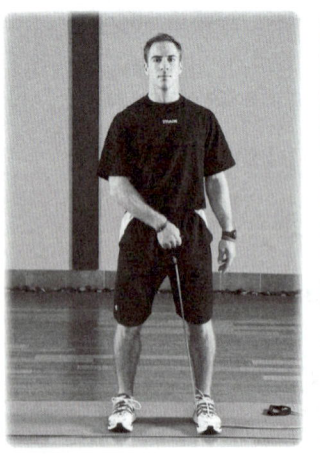

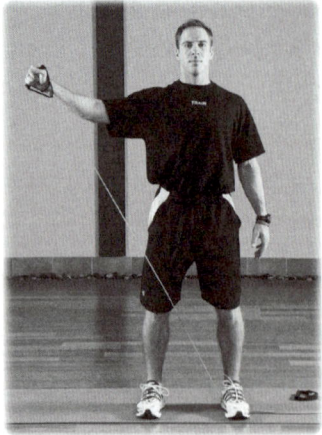

Too hard? Use lighter resistance tubing.
Too easy? Use heavier resistance tubing.

Resistance band and tube workout

6 | Squat

Reps: 8–12
Sets: 1–3
Intensity: Moderate
Tempo: 4-4
Rest: 30–90 seconds between sets

Starting position: Stand on the resistance tubing with your feet hip-width apart. Bring the resistance tubing up behind your shoulders so that you are holding the handles on top of your shoulders with your palms facing forward.

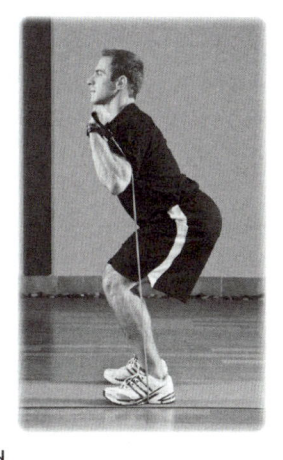

Movement: Hinge forward at the hips and bend your knees to lower your buttocks toward the floor as if sitting down in a chair. Throughout the movement, press your weight back into your heels and keep the handles on top of your shoulders. Return to the starting position.

Tips and techniques:
- Keep your hips, knees, and feet aligned and pointing front.
- When squatting, your knees should extend no farther than your toes.
- Stop with your buttocks above knee level.

Too hard? Perform a shallower squat. Use lighter resistance tubing.
Too easy? Use heavier resistance tubing. Also, pause and hold for 4 counts while squatting, before returning to the starting position.

7 | Traveling side squat

Reps: 8–12
Sets: 1–3
Intensity: Moderate to high
Tempo: 2-2
Rest: 30–90 seconds

Starting position: Stand with your feet slightly apart and clasp your hands loosely in front of your chest. Place a resistance band around both thighs just above your knees.

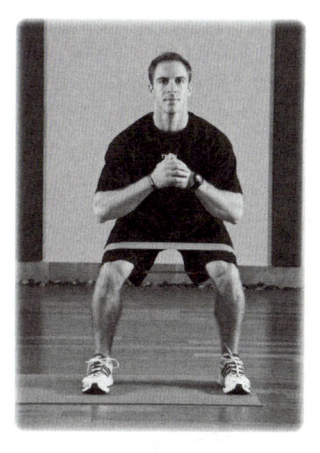

Movement: Step out to your right side as you bend your knees and lower to a squat position. Rise up as you bring your legs together just enough to maintain resistance on the band. Do 4–6 traveling squats to the right, then 4–6 to the left.

Tips and techniques:
- Keep your hips, knees, and toes all pointing forward.
- Drop your buttocks no lower than your knees.

Too hard? Use a lighter resistance band or no band.
Too easy? Lower the resistance band to your ankles.

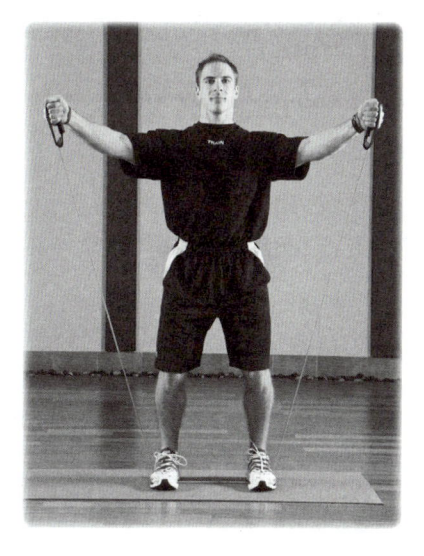

8 | V-raise

Reps: 8–12
Sets: 1–3
Intensity: Moderate to high
Tempo: 3-3
Rest: 30–90 seconds

Starting position: Stand with the resistance tubing under your feet. Position your feet hip-width apart and place your hands at your sides with thumbs pointing forward as you hold the handles.

Movement: Squeeze your shoulder blades together while you slowly lift your arms toward the two front corners of the room, creating a V as you raise the resistance tubing. Go no higher than your shoulders. Slowly return to the starting position.

Tips and techniques:
- Keep your wrists firm, maintaining a straight line from your elbow to your knuckles, and elbows soft (not locked) throughout the movement.
- Keep your shoulders down and back.
- Exhale as you lift.

Too hard? Use lighter resistance tubing.
Too easy? Use heavier resistance tubing.

Ball workout

By using a stability ball and a medicine ball, this workout enhances balance while tuning up strength. Ironically, a stability ball introduces an element of instability, engaging a bevy of core muscles to hold you steady that wouldn't be in use if you stood on a flat surface. Another nice variation in several of the exercises is a torso rotation that works core muscles used in many sports, including golf, kayaking, tennis, and swimming. Remember to include a warm-up and cool-down, too.

Equipment:
- Stability ball
- Medicine ball
- Mat, towels, or carpet for comfort during floor exercises

1 | Knee lift with rotation

Reps: 8–12
Sets: 1–3
Intensity: Moderate
Tempo: 2-2-2-2
Rest: 30–90 seconds between sets

Starting position: Sit on the stability ball with your feet hip-width apart. Hold a medicine ball with both hands at waist level.

Movement: Lift your right knee toward the ceiling. Squeezing the medicine ball with both hands to engage your core muscles, slowly rotate your torso to the right. Slowly rotate back to the center, then lower your leg to the floor. Repeat on the left side for one full rep.

Tips and techniques:
- Keep your movements slow and controlled.
- Maintain neutral posture.
- Keep your chest lifted and shoulders down and back.

Too hard? Keep both feet on the floor and perform only the torso rotation.
Too easy? Use a heavier medicine ball.

2 | Pull-over on stability ball

Reps: 8–12
Sets: 1–3
Intensity: Moderate
Tempo: 4-4
Rest: 30–90 seconds between sets

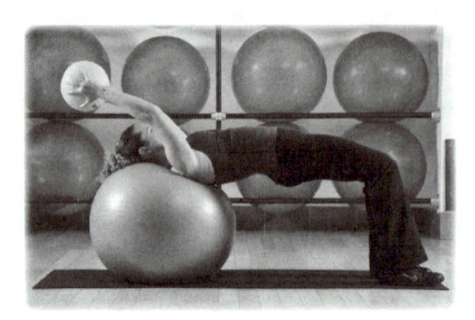

Starting position: Sit on the stability ball holding a medicine ball against your stomach. Roll downward until the back of your head and shoulders are on the stability ball. Position your feet shoulder-width apart and lift your hips and buttocks up in the bridge position. Align your knees directly over your ankles. Now lift the medicine ball toward the ceiling above your chest.

Movement: Keeping your arms fully extended, lower the medicine ball toward the wall behind you. Then lift the medicine ball back toward the ceiling above your chest.

Tips and techniques:
- Tighten your abdominal muscles as you return to the starting position.
- Keep your shoulders, hips, and knees in a straight line.
- Keep your knees in line directly over your ankles.

Too hard? Perform the exercise lying on your back on the floor.
Too easy? Use a heavier medicine ball.

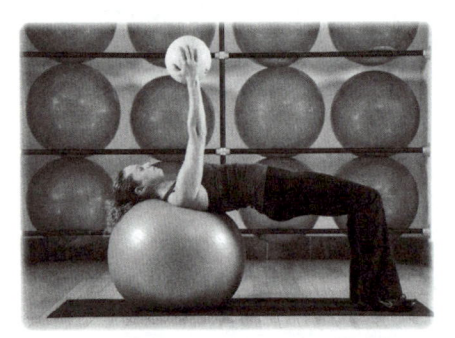

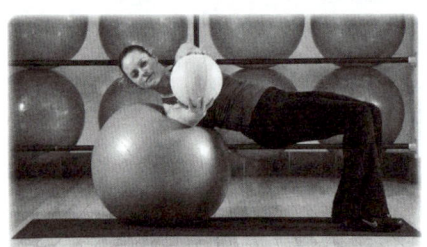

3 | Torso rotation with medicine ball

Reps: 8–12
Sets: 1–3
Intensity: Moderate to high
Tempo: 4-4
Rest: 30–90 seconds between sets

Starting position: Sit on the stability ball holding a medicine ball with both hands. Roll downward until the back of your head and shoulders are on the stability ball. Position your feet shoulder-width apart and lift your hips and buttocks up in the bridge position. Align your knees directly over your ankles. Now lift the medicine ball toward the ceiling above your chest.

Movement: Keeping your arms extended, rotate your head, arms, and torso toward the right wall. Return to the starting position. Repeat to the left for one full rep.

Tips and techniques:
- Engage your core by squeezing your buttocks and tightening your abdominal muscles.
- As you rotate your torso, your head and upper shoulder will come off the ball.
- Keep your lower body still throughout the movement.

Too hard? Use a lighter medicine ball.
Too easy? Use a heavier medicine ball.

Ball workout

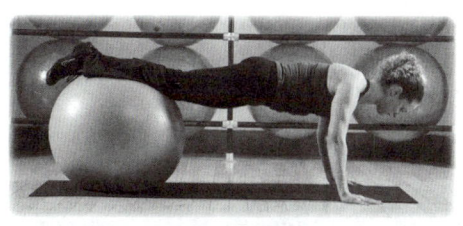

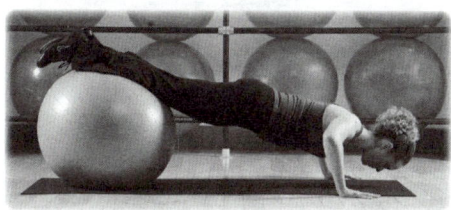

4 | Push-up on stability ball

Reps: 8–12
Sets: 1–3
Intensity: Moderate to high
Tempo: 3-1
Rest: 30–90 seconds between sets

Starting position: Lie on your stomach on a stability ball with your hands on the floor in front of you. While contracting your abdominal muscles, walk your hands out until you are in a comfortable plank position with your legs on the ball and your hands directly under your shoulders.

Movement: Bend your elbows to slowly lower your chest toward the floor. Straighten your arms to return to the starting position.

Tips and techniques:
- Keep your head and spine neutral.
- Lead with your chest (not your head) as you lower yourself into the push-up.
- Inhale as you lower; exhale as you lift.

Too hard? Walk your hands out a shorter distance to position the ball higher on your legs before doing push-ups.
Too easy? While maintaining correct alignment with your hands directly under your shoulders, walk your hands farther away from the ball before doing push-ups.

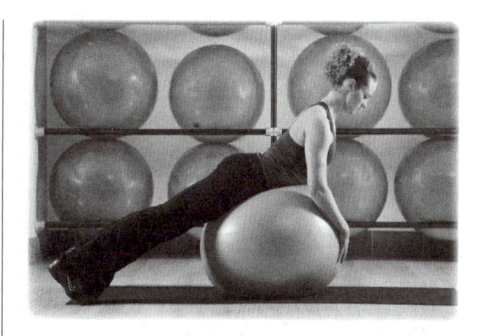

5 | Back extension on stability ball

Reps: 8–12
Sets: 1–3
Intensity: Moderate
Tempo: 4-4
Rest: 30–90 seconds between sets

Starting position: Lie on your stomach on a stability ball, keeping the ball centered under your waist. Wrap your forearms around the front of the ball. Position your feet about hip-width apart and lift your knees off the floor so that you are balancing on the stability ball with the balls of your feet pressing into the floor.

Movement: Slowly lift your chest off the stability ball until your body is in a straight line from the top of your head to your tailbone. Do not overextend. Slowly return to the starting position.

Tips and techniques:
- Keep your neck neutral throughout the movement.
- Use your spine muscles, not your arms, to lift your torso.
- Exhale as you lift.

Too hard? Keep your knees on the floor and lift your chest less.
Too easy? Do the exercise with your hands clasped and placed gently on your forehead and your elbows out to the sides.

6 | Leg curl on stability ball

Reps: 8–12
Sets: 1–3
Intensity: Moderate to high
Tempo: 2-2
Rest: 30–90 seconds between sets

Starting position: Lie on your back with both legs extended and your feet on top of the stability ball. Rest your arms on the floor at your sides and lift your hips.

Movement: Bend your knees to pull the ball in toward your buttocks until your feet are flat on the ball. Keeping your hips raised, return to the starting position.

Tips and techniques:
- Keep your spine neutral.
- Tighten your abdominal and buttock muscles.
- Keep your knees soft (not locked) when straightening your legs.

Too hard? Perform the exercise with your buttocks on the floor.
Too easy? Cross your arms over your chest before starting the leg curl.

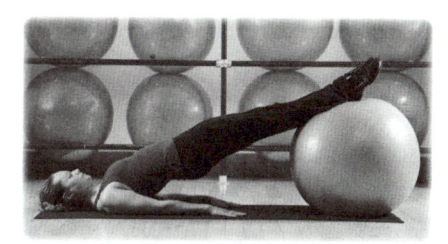

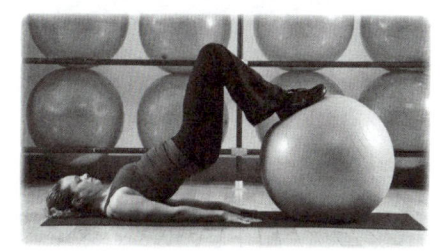

www.health.harvard.edu

Ball workout

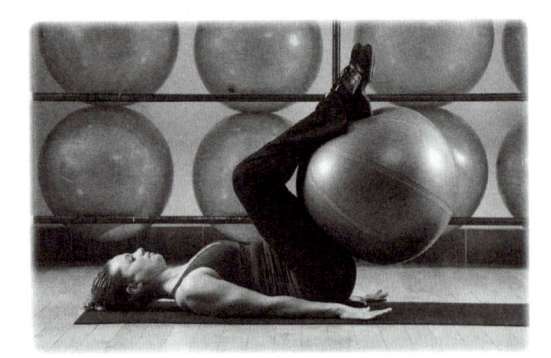

7 | Reverse curl with stability ball

Reps: 8–12
Sets: 1–3
Intensity: Moderate
Tempo: 2-2-2
Rest: 30–90 seconds between sets

Starting position: Lie on your back with your knees bent over the stability ball and heels gripping it. Place your arms on the floor at your sides.

Movement: Grip the ball with your heels as you tighten your abdominal muscles to lift your hips and the ball off the floor. Pause, then return to the starting position.

Tips and techniques:
- In the starting position, keep your knees directly over your hips.
- Exhale and contract your abdominal muscles as you curl your hips toward your ribs.

Too hard? Press your palms down into the floor to help lift your hips and stabilize the movement.
Too easy? Place your hands gently behind your head with your elbows out to the sides. Lift your head and shoulders off the floor as you do the reverse curl.

8 | Wall squat with stability ball and medicine ball

Reps: 8–12
Sets: 1–3
Intensity: Moderate
Tempo: 4-4
Rest: 30–90 seconds between sets

Starting position: Stand up straight and place the stability ball between the back of your waist and the wall. Walk your feet out about 18 to 24 inches. Hold a medicine ball close to the front of your waist.

Movement: As you lift the medicine ball to chest level, slowly bend your knees and hips into a squat as if you were sitting down in a chair. Stop before your buttocks reach knee level. Straighten your legs as you return to the starting position.

Tips and techniques:
- Maintain neutral posture with chin parallel to the floor, chest lifted, and shoulders down and back.
- Keep your knees aligned over your ankles and pointing forward as you squat.
- Exhale as you return to the starting position.

Too hard? Do a smaller squat.
Too easy? Hold the squat for 8 counts. Or do single leg squats with one foot lifted off the floor, then repeat on the other side.

SUPERSET ME

Want to try supersets? Combine these:
- Pull-over on stability ball + Torso rotation with medicine ball
- Push-up on stability ball + Back extension on stability ball

See "Supersets," page 17, for more information.

Mixed workout: Bosu, weights and medicine ball

Tired of the same-old, same-old? Mix it up in a full-body workout that improves strength and stability using a Bosu, weights, and a medicine ball. Bosu moves are particularly good for strengthening your core because instability prompts you to tighten your abdominal and back muscles to hold yourself steady while you do the exercises. Remember to bracket your workout with a warm-up and cool-down.

Equipment:
- Bosu • Weights • Medicine ball • Mat, towels, or carpet for comfort during floor exercises

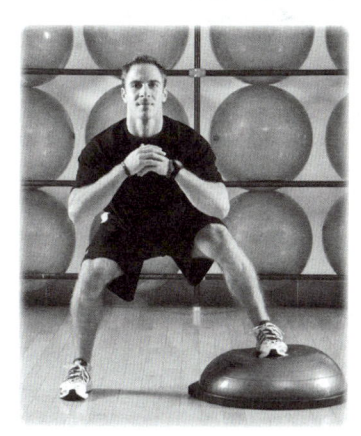

1 | Squat from Bosu

Reps: 8–12 on each side
Sets: 1–3
Intensity: Moderate to high
Tempo: 4-4
Rest: 30–90 seconds between sets

Starting position: Stand with both feet on top of the Bosu. Extend your arms out in front of your chest with your elbows bent and hands together.

Movement: Tighten your abdominal muscles. Step off the Bosu directly to your right, hinging forward at the hips and bending both knees to lower your buttocks toward the floor as if sitting down in a chair. Go no farther than knee level. Return to the starting position. Finish all reps before repeating with the leg positions reversed. This is one complete set.

Tips and techniques:
- When lowering yourself into the squat, bend from the hip and press your weight back into your heels.
- Maintain neutral posture, chest lifted, shoulders down and back.

Too hard? Perform on the floor.
Too easy? Add a knee lift as you return to the top of the Bosu.

SUPERSET ME

Want to try supersets? Combine these:
- Squat on Bosu with medicine ball + Lunge from Bosu
- Opposite arm and leg raise on Bosu + Plank on Bosu

See "Supersets," page 17, for more information.

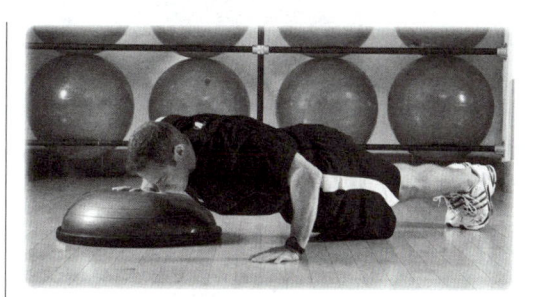

2 | Push-up on Bosu

Reps: 8–12 on each side
Sets: 1–3
Intensity: Moderate to high
Tempo: 2-2
Rest: 30–90 seconds between sets

Starting position: Position yourself at the top of a push-up with both arms straight, right hand on top of the Bosu and left hand on the floor, shoulder-width apart. Extend your legs with feet flexed and toes touching the floor. Tighten your abdominal muscles throughout to help maintain a neutral spine and keep your body aligned from the top of your head to your heels.

Movement: Bend your elbows to lower your chest toward the Bosu and floor. Straighten your elbows as you push up to return to the starting position. Finish all reps before repeating with your left hand on top of the Bosu. This is one complete set.

Tips and techniques:
- Keep your shoulders down and back with your neck and spine in neutral position.
- Keep your elbows slightly bent at the top of the push-up.
- Exhale as you return to the starting position.

Too hard? Do the exercise with both knees bent and on the floor.
Too easy? Lift one leg in the air as you do the exercise.

Mixed workout

3 | Lunge from Bosu

Reps: 8–12
Sets: 1–3
Intensity: Moderate to high
Tempo: 4-4
Rest: 30–90 seconds between sets

Starting position: Stand with both feet on top of the Bosu, elbows bent and hands in front of your chest. Lift your chest and keep your shoulders down and back.

Movement: Step backward off the Bosu, placing the ball of your right foot on the floor behind you. Slowly sink into the reverse lunge position by bending your knees until your right knee points to the floor and your left knee aligns over your ankle. Keep your torso straight as you do this and evenly distribute your weight over both legs. Return to the starting position by bringing your right foot back up on top of the Bosu. Exhale as you lift up. Repeat with the left leg for one full rep.

Tips and techniques:
- Keep your chest lifted and maintain a neutral spine.
- Keep your knees in line with your ankles.

Too hard? Do reverse lunges on the floor, or do a shallower lunge.
Too easy? Before bringing your rear leg back to the starting position on the Bosu, add a knee lift.

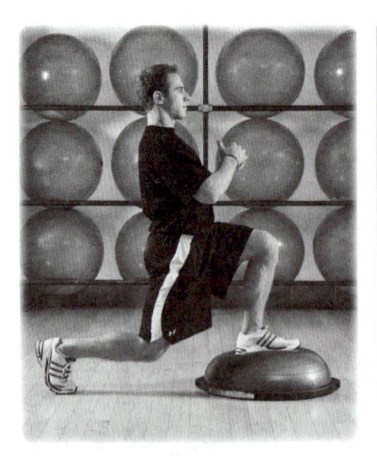

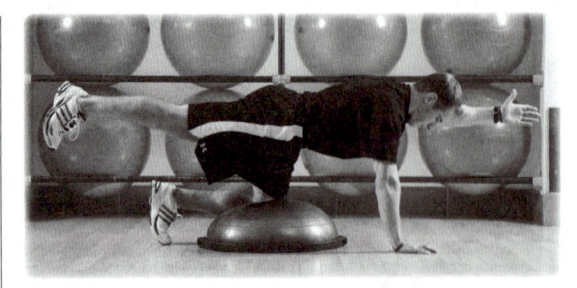

4 | Opposite arm and leg raise on Bosu

Reps: 8–12
Sets: 1–3
Intensity: Moderate
Tempo: 2-4-2
Rest: 30–90 seconds between sets

Starting position: Kneel with knees on the Bosu and toes resting on the floor behind you. Place both hands on the floor in front of you, directly under your shoulders. Keep your head and spine neutral.

Movement: Slowly extend your right leg off the floor behind you as you simultaneously reach out in front of you with your left arm, thumb up. Keep your hips and shoulders squared while trying to bring the leg and arm parallel to the floor. Pause, then slowly return to the starting position. Repeat with the other leg and arm for one full rep.

Tips and techniques:
- Tighten your abdominal muscles during the exercise to engage your core.
- Imagine someone pulling your arm and leg to lengthen your torso. Keep your head and neck neutral.

Too hard? Perform on the floor or try lifting only an arm, or a leg.
Too easy? Hold small hand weights.

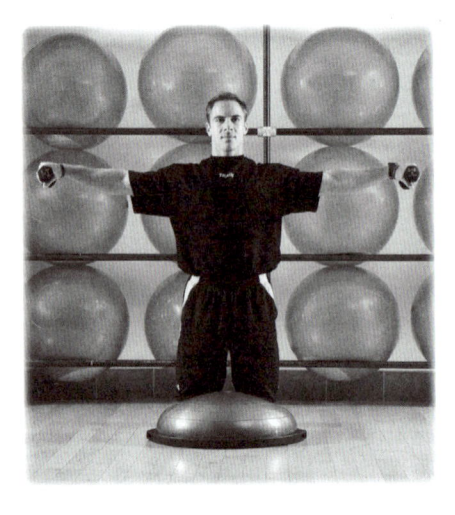

5 | Lateral raise kneeling on Bosu

Reps: 8–12
Sets: 1–3
Intensity: Moderate to high
Tempo: 3-1
Rest: 30–90 seconds between sets

Starting position: Kneel on the Bosu with both knees, resting your toes on the floor behind you. Maintain a neutral spine. Hold weights with your hands at your sides and thumbs pointing forward.

Movement: Lift your chest and press your shoulders down and back as you slowly raise your arms to the side to the height of your shoulders. Slowly return to the starting position.

Tips and techniques:
- Tighten your abdominal muscles and squeeze your buttocks to engage your core.
- Keep your elbows slightly bent throughout the movement.
- Exhale as you lift.

Too hard? Use a lighter weight.
Too easy? Lift both toes off the floor or hold a heavier weight.

Mixed workout

6 | Squat on Bosu with medicine ball

Reps: 8–12
Sets: 1–3
Intensity: High
Tempo: 4-4
Rest: 30–90 seconds between sets

Starting position: Stand up straight on top of the Bosu holding a medicine ball close to your waist. Lift your chest and roll your shoulders down and back.

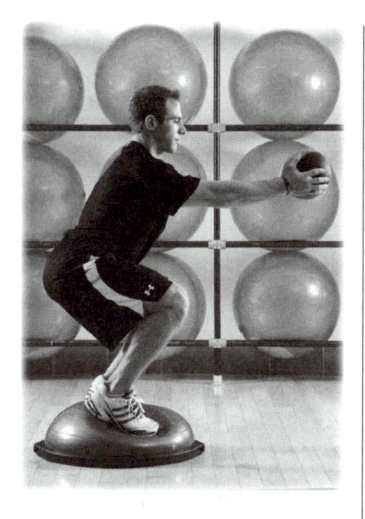

Movement: Slowly bend your knees and hinge forward at the hips to lower your buttocks as if you are sitting down in a chair; stop with your buttocks above knee level. As you squat, extend your arms out in front of your chest holding the medicine ball. As you return to the starting position, bring the medicine ball back to your waist. Maintain neutral posture with chest lifted and shoulders down and back.

Tips and techniques:
- Keep your hips, knees, and toes pointing forward.
- Keep your knees in line with your ankles, extending no farther than your toes.
- Exhale as you lift up.

Too hard? Do the exercise without the medicine ball or try doing it on the floor.
Too easy? Use a heavier medicine ball.

7 | Biceps curl on Bosu

Reps: 8–12
Sets: 1–3
Intensity: Moderate to high
Tempo: 1-3
Rest: 30–90 seconds between sets

Starting position: Stand up straight on top of the Bosu, holding weights at your sides with your palms pointing forward.

Movement: Tighten your abdominal and buttock muscles to engage your core for stability. Bend your elbows to lift the weights up to the front of your shoulders. Slowly lower them to the starting position.

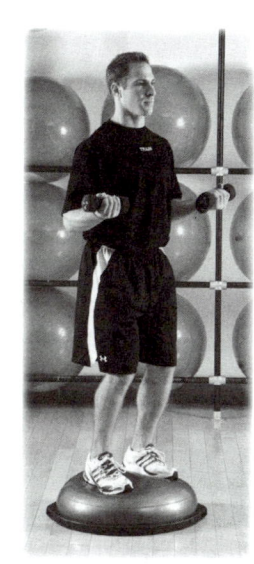

Tips and techniques:
- Keep your shoulders still, down, and back.
- Keep your wrists neutral and elbows stationary at the sides of your ribs throughout the movement.
- Exhale as you lift.

Too hard? Use lighter weights, or do the exercise standing on the floor.
Too easy? Use heavier weights.

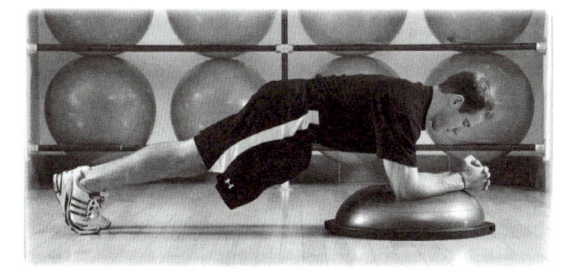

8 | Plank on Bosu

Reps: 4–6
Sets: 1
Intensity: High
Hold: 15–60 seconds
Rest: 30–90 seconds between reps

Starting position: Place your forearms on top of the Bosu with your elbows under your shoulders, hands loosely clasped, and knees on the floor with your toes tucked under.

Movement: Tighten your abdominal muscles as you lift your knees off the floor and extend your lower body into a full plank position. Check that your shoulders are directly over your elbows. Maintain neutral alignment from the top of your head to your heels. Hold for 15–60 seconds, then return to the starting position.

Tips and techniques:
- Keep your abdominal muscles tightened throughout the movement.
- Maintain a neutral spine.
- Keep your shoulders down and back to stabilize the shoulder blades.

Too hard? Do the exercise on the floor without the Bosu.
Too easy? Lift one leg off the floor during the exercise. Finish all reps before repeating with the leg positions reversed. This is one complete set.

THE WORKOUTS

Core workout

Six-pack abs are the holy grail for core workout enthusiasts. While that ripped look still goes far on the beach, you'll be better served once you shake the sand off your feet if all of your core muscles are strong and well-balanced. Strong core muscles support your back. By performing this workout regularly, you may save yourself backaches and possible injuries—and you'll look great!

Equipment:
- Medicine ball
- Mat, towels, or carpet for comfort during floor exercises

1 | Alternating forward lunge with medicine ball

Reps: 8–12
Sets: 1–3
Intensity: Moderate to high
Tempo: 2-2
Rest: 30–90 seconds between sets

Starting position: Stand up straight holding the medicine ball at your waist.

Movement: Step forward on your right leg, keeping the medicine ball close to your waist as you bend your knees and sink into a lunge. Your right knee should align over your ankle and your left knee should point to the floor. Return to the starting position. Repeat the movement with the left leg forward. This completes one rep.

Tips and techniques:
- Maintain a neutral spine throughout.
- In the lunge position, align the knee of the forward leg over the ankle. The heel of the rear leg lifts off the floor and that knee bends enough to form a straight line from shoulder to hip to knee.
- Exhale as you return to the starting position.

Too hard? Do the exercise without the medicine ball, or do a shallower lunge.
Too easy? Lift the knee of the forward leg toward the ceiling as you return to the starting position.

SUPERSET ME

Want to try supersets? Combine these:
- Alternating forward lunge with medicine ball + Walking lunge with diagonal reach
- Back plank + Bicycle

See "Supersets," page 17, for more information.

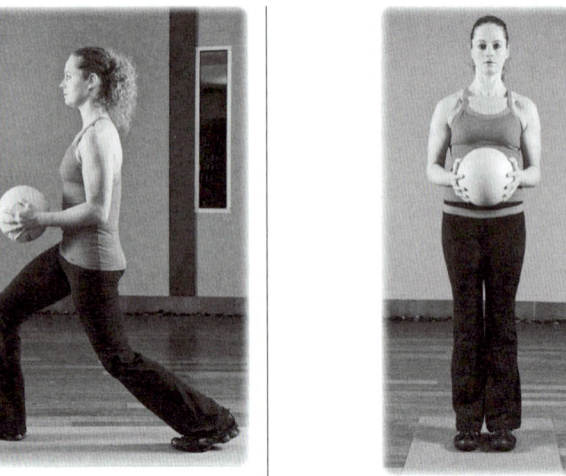

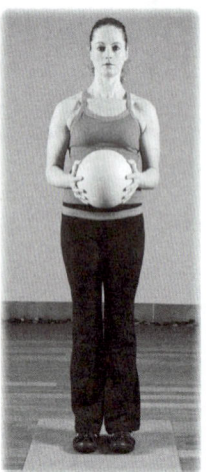

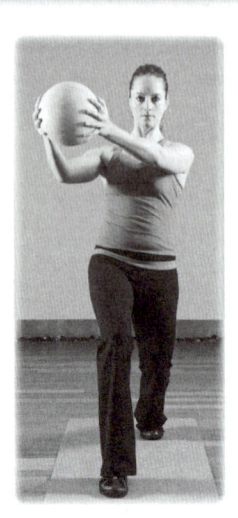

2 | Walking lunge with diagonal reach

Reps: 8–12
Sets: 1–3
Intensity: Moderate to high
Tempo: 2-2-2-2
Rest: 30–90 seconds between sets

Starting position: Stand up straight with your feet a few inches apart, holding the medicine ball at your waist.

Movement: Step forward on your right leg into the lunge position as you extend your arms and lift the medicine ball diagonally up to the right as high as your shoulder. Then bring your left foot to your right foot while lowering the medicine ball diagonally down to your waist to return to the starting position. Repeat the lunge with the left leg as you extend your arms and lift the medicine ball diagonally up to the left as high as your shoulder. Then bring your right foot to your left foot while lowering the medicine ball diagonally down to your waist. This completes one rep.

Tips and techniques:
- Maintain a neutral spine throughout the lunge.
- In the lunge position, align the knee of the forward leg over the ankle. The heel of the rear leg lifts off the floor and that knee bends enough to form a straight line from shoulder to hip to knee.
- Notice the tempo is slow to help you stay in control during each part of the movement.

Too hard? Do the exercise without the medicine ball, or do a shallower lunge.
Too easy? Hold a heavier medicine ball.

32   Workout Workbook   www.health.harvard.edu

Core workout

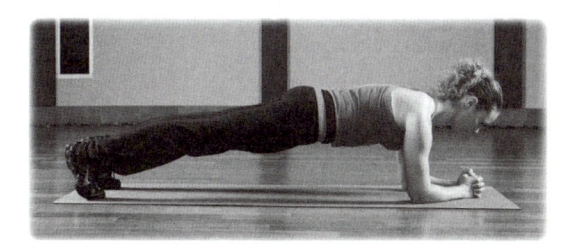

3 | Front plank

Reps: 2–4
Sets: 1
Intensity: Moderate to high
Hold: 15–60 seconds
Rest: 30–90 seconds between reps

Starting position: Start on your hands and knees.

Movement: Tighten your abdominal muscles and lower your upper body to your forearms, clasping your hands together and aligning your shoulders directly over your elbows. Extend both legs with your feet flexed and toes touching the floor so that you balance your body in a line like a plank. Hold.

Tips and techniques:
- Keep your neck and spine neutral during the plank, not curving upward or downward.
- Keep your shoulders down and back.
- Breathe comfortably.

Too hard? Put your knees on the floor instead of extending your legs.
Too easy? While holding your body in a line like a plank, lift your right foot and move it to the side six inches, tap the floor, and move it back to the center. Lift your left foot and move it to the side six inches, tap the floor, and move it back to the center. Continue for 15 to 60 seconds.

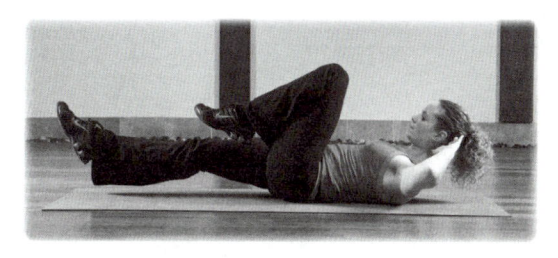

4 | Bicycle

Reps: 8–12
Sets: 1–3
Intensity: Moderate to high
Tempo: 2-2
Rest: 30–90 seconds between sets

Starting position: Lie on your back with your left leg extended on the floor. Bring your right knee in toward your chest. Place hands lightly behind your head.

Movement: Exhale as you tighten your abdominal muscles. Lift your head and shoulders off the floor. Extend your right leg, a few inches off the floor, and bring your left knee in toward your chest. Then extend your left leg, a few inches off the floor, and bring your right knee in toward your chest to complete one rep.

Tips and techniques:
- Engage your core by tightening your abdominal muscles before lifting your shoulders.
- Avoid pulling on your head and neck.

Too hard? Put your fingertips on the floor, behind your waist, before starting the bicycle.
Too easy? Cross your arms over your chest before starting the bicycle, or increase the number of reps.

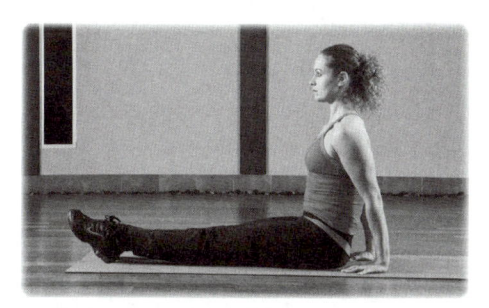

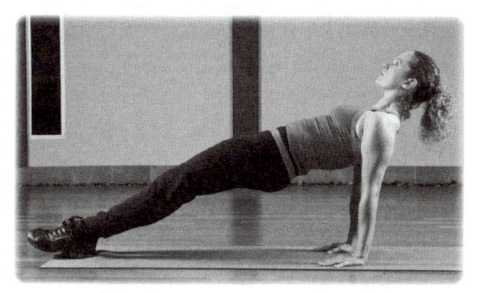

5 | Back plank

Reps: 2–4
Sets: 1
Intensity: Moderate to high
Hold: 15–60 seconds
Rest: 30–90 seconds between reps

Starting position: Sit up straight on the floor with your legs extended. Place your hands directly below your shoulders with fingertips pointing forward.

Movement: Tighten your abdominal and buttock muscles as you lift your hips up to form a straight line from head to toe.

Tips and techniques:
- Maintain a neutral neck and spine.
- Keep your shoulders down and back.

Too hard? Lean back, balancing on your forearms with your elbows directly below your shoulders.
Too easy? While in the plank position, lift one leg and then the other.

www.health.harvard.edu   Workout Workbook   33

Core workout

6 | Hip-up

Reps: 8–12
Sets: 1–3
Intensity: Moderate to high
Tempo: 2-2
Rest: 30–90 seconds between sets

Starting position: Lie on your back with both legs hinged at the hips and extended up toward the ceiling. Place your hands at your sides.

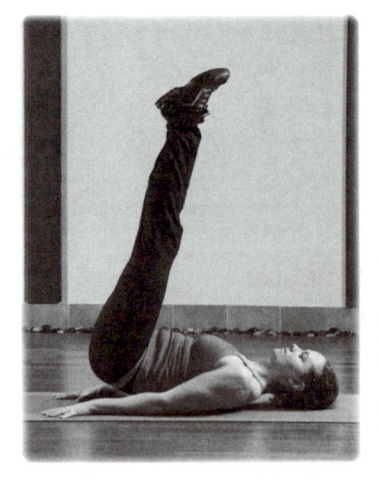

Movement: Tighten your abdominal and buttock muscles as you lift your hips a few inches off the floor. Return to the starting position.

Tips and techniques:
- Try to lift your legs and hips straight up toward the ceiling slowly, with control to avoid a rocking motion.
- If necessary, place your hands on the floor to assist you and maintain balance.

Too hard? Start with 4–6 repetitions.
Too easy? Pause for one count at the top of the lift.

7 | Plié with medicine ball

Reps: 8–12
Sets: 1–3
Intensity: Moderate
Tempo: 2-2
Rest: 30–90 seconds between sets

Starting position: Stand up straight with your feet placed slightly wider than your hips. Turn your toes outward (rotating from the hip) as far as is comfortable. Keep your knees, ankles, and toes aligned. Hold the medicine ball with your arms extended down toward the floor.

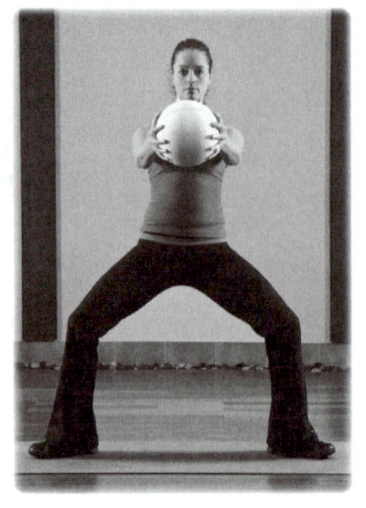

Movement: Bend your knees as you lift the medicine ball directly out in front of your chest. Stop before your buttocks reach knee level. Return to the starting position.

Tips and techniques:
- Keep your torso upright and shoulders down and back.
- Squeeze your inner thighs as you straighten your legs to return to the starting position.

Too hard? Do the plié without the medicine ball, or bend your knees less as you plié.
Too easy? Hold a heavier ball or lift the ball directly overhead.

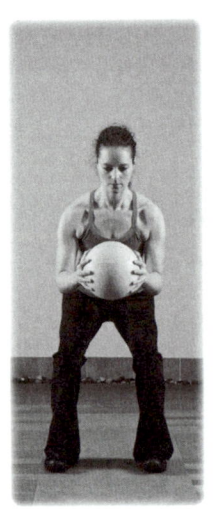

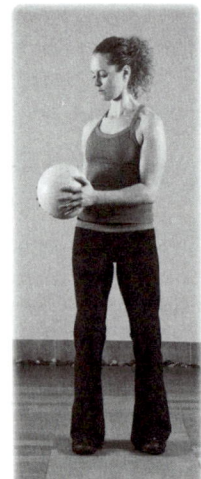

8 | Squat with rotation and medicine ball

Reps: 8–12
Sets: 1–3
Intensity: Moderate
Tempo: 2-2-2-2
Rest: 30–90 seconds between sets

Starting position: Stand up straight with your feet hip-width apart, holding a medicine ball at your waist.

Movement: Hinge forward at the hips and squat as if sitting down in a chair. Stop with your buttocks above knee level. Return to the starting position. Bending your knees slightly, rotate your torso to the right, then return to center. Repeat movements on the left side for one full rep.

Tips and techniques:
- Hinge forward from your hips and press your weight back into your heels as you squat. Keep your chest lifted and your shoulders down and back.
- Keep your hips and knees pointing to the front while rotating from the waist.

Too hard? Just do squats to each side without the rotation.
Too easy? As you rotate to the right, lift your right knee. As you rotate to the left, lift your left knee.

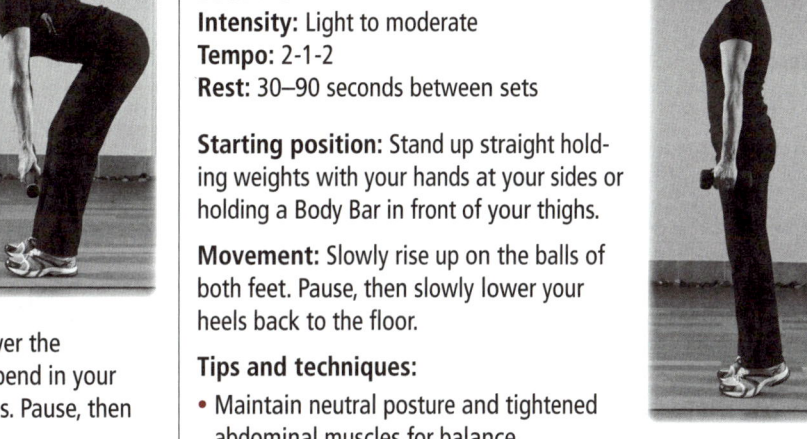

Split strength workout: Lower body

The large muscles of your lower body—quads, hamstrings, and gluteus muscles—power you through your daily rounds. This workout strengthens and tones major and minor players in the lower-body league. Try the Body Bar in place of hand weights for a change. For a full strength routine, pair these exercises with the upper-body exercises on page 38. You can blend all of the exercises into a single workout or do the lower body one day and the upper body on another. Rest 48 hours between lower-body strength sessions, and be sure you bracket your workout with a warm-up and cool-down.

Equipment:
• Hand weights • Ankle weights (optional) • Resistance band • Stability ball • Body Bar (optional) • Mat, towels, or carpet for comfort during floor exercises

1 | Dead lift with weights

Reps: 8–12   **Sets:** 1–3
Intensity: Moderate to high
Tempo: 2-1-2
Rest: 30–90 seconds between sets

Starting position: Stand up straight with your feet hip-width apart, holding hand weights or a Body Bar with your palms facing the front of your thighs. Bend your knees slightly. Keep your neck and spine neutral and shoulders down and back.

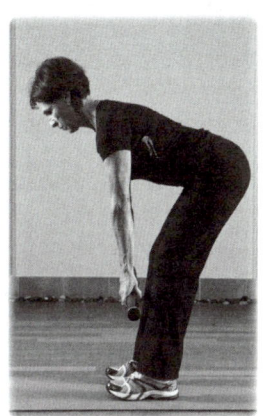

Movement: Bend forward at the hips as you lower the weights toward the floor, maintaining the slight bend in your knees and neutral spine. Stop just past your knees. Pause, then exhale as you return to the starting position.

Tips and techniques:
• Keep the movement slow and controlled.
• As you bend forward, keep your upper body in a straight line from the top of your head to your tailbone.
• Exhale as you lift.

Too hard? Use lighter weights.
Too easy? Use heavier weights.

2 | Heel raise with weights

Reps: 8–12
Sets: 1–3
Intensity: Light to moderate
Tempo: 2-1-2
Rest: 30–90 seconds between sets

Starting position: Stand up straight holding weights with your hands at your sides or holding a Body Bar in front of your thighs.

Movement: Slowly rise up on the balls of both feet. Pause, then slowly lower your heels back to the floor.

Tips and techniques:
• Maintain neutral posture and tightened abdominal muscles for balance.
• As you lift, keep your ankles firm to avoid rolling to the outside of your foot.
• Exhale as you lift up.

Too hard? Do the exercise without weights.
Too easy? Try the exercise while standing on only your right leg. Finish all reps before repeating with your left leg. This is one complete set.

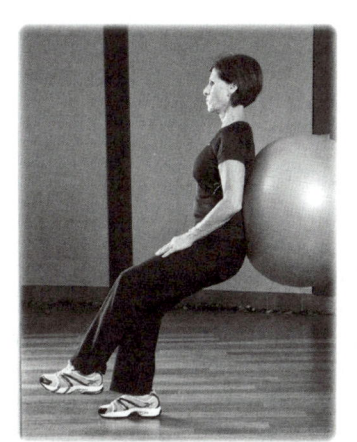

3 | Single leg squat with stability ball

Reps: 8–12 on each side
Sets: 1–3
Intensity: Moderate to high
Tempo: 2-2
Rest: 30–90 seconds between sets

Starting position: Stand with your back to a wall and position a stability ball behind you at your waist. Walk your feet a few steps forward so that your knees will align over your ankles when bent. Put your arms at your sides or hands on your thighs, and lift your left leg a few inches off the floor.

Movement: Keep your back pressing against the stability ball and tighten your buttocks as you slowly bend your right knee into a squat as if sitting down in a chair. Stop with your buttocks above knee level. Press down into your right heel while returning to the starting position. Exhale as you lift up. Finish all reps before repeating with the leg positions reversed. This is one complete set.

Tips and techniques:
• Maintain neutral posture with chin parallel to the floor.
• Keep your knee aligned over your ankle and your buttocks above the level of your bent knee.

Too hard? Do the squat with both feet on the floor and sink down a shorter distance.
Too easy? Hold hand weights.

Split strength workout: Lower body

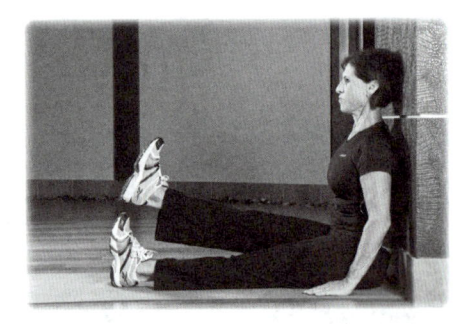

4 | Seated leg lift

Reps: 8–12 on each side
Sets: 1–3
Intensity: Moderate to high
Tempo: 2-1-2
Rest: 30–90 seconds between sets

Starting position: Sit on the floor with your back to a wall and your legs extended in front of you. Rest your hands by your hips on the floor.

Movement: Contract your thigh muscles and lift your right leg in the air. Pause, then lower the leg to the floor. Finish all reps before repeating with the leg positions reversed. This is one complete set.

Tips and techniques:
- Make sure your buttocks are against the wall.
- Maintain neutral posture with shoulders down and back.
- Exhale as you lift.

Too hard? Lie on your back with your right leg extended and your left knee bent with the foot on the floor. Lift your right leg. Pause, then lower the leg. Finish all reps before repeating with the left leg. This is one complete set.

Too easy? Add an ankle weight.

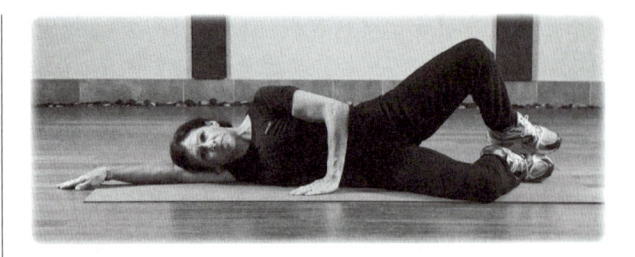

5 | Clam

Reps: 8–12 on each side
Sets: 1–3
Intensity: Light to moderate
Tempo: 2-1-2
Rest: 30–90 seconds between sets

Starting position: Lie on your right side, knees bent so your heels are in line with your buttocks. Rest your head on your right arm on the floor.

Movement: Keep your feet together as you lift your left knee up toward the ceiling. Pause, then return to the starting position. Finish all reps before repeating on the other side. This is one complete set.

Tips and techniques:
- Throughout the movement, keep your hips stacked and still as if you were lying against a wall.
- Lift your top knee up as high as possible without letting your hip move.
- Exhale as you lift.

Too hard? Lift your top knee less high.

Too easy? Place a resistance band around your upper thighs above your knees, or increase the number of reps.

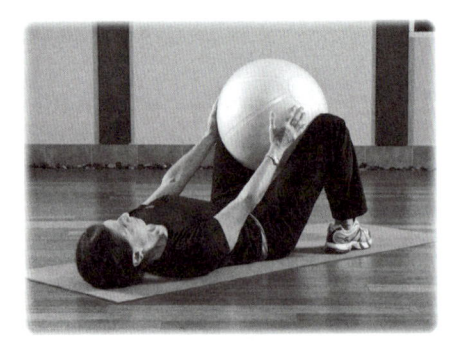

6 | Inner thigh squeeze with stability ball

Reps: 8–12
Sets: 1–3
Intensity: Light to moderate
Tempo: 2-5-2
Rest: 30–90 seconds between sets

Starting position: Lie on your back with your knees bent and feet on the floor. Place the stability ball between your knees. Put your hands on the ball for support.

Movement: Tighten your inner thigh and buttock muscles as you squeeze the stability ball between your knees. Hold for 5 seconds, then release to the starting position.

Tips and techniques:
- Maintain neutral posture without arching or flexing your back.
- Breathe comfortably.
- Exhale as you squeeze the ball.

Too hard? Squeeze more gently, then release.

Too easy? Lift both feet up toward the ceiling and place the stability ball between your lower legs and feet. Put your hands on the outside of your legs for support. Squeeze, hold, then release to the starting position.

Split strength workout: Lower body

7 | Traveling side squat

Reps: 8–12
Sets: 1–3
Intensity: Moderate to high
Tempo: 2-2
Rest: 30–90 seconds between sets

Starting position: Stand with your feet slightly apart. Place a resistance band around both thighs just above your knees.

Movement: Step out to your right side as you bend your knees and lower your buttocks to a squat position as if sitting down in a chair. Rise up while bringing your legs together just enough to maintain resistance on the band so that it doesn't fall off. Do 4–6 traveling squats to the right, then 4–6 to the left.

Tips and techniques:
- Keep your hips, knees, and toes all pointing forward.
- Stop with your buttocks above knee level.
- Exhale as you lift up from the squat.

Too hard? Use a lighter resistance band or no band.
Too easy? Place the resistance band around your ankles.

SUPERSET ME

Want to try supersets? Combine these:
- Dead lift with weights + Single leg squat with stability ball
- Plié with weights + Heel raise with weight

See "Supersets," page 17, for more information.

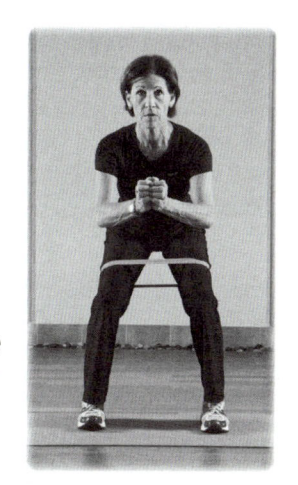

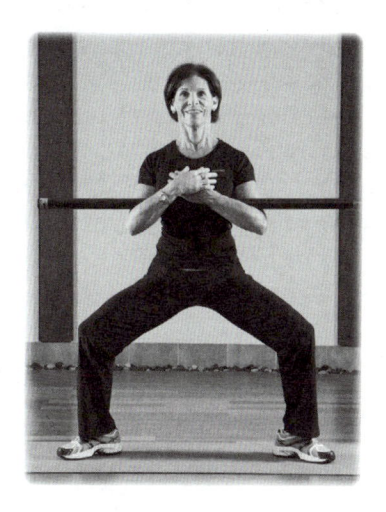

8 | Plié with weights

Reps: 8–12
Sets: 1–3
Intensity: Moderate
Tempo: 2-2
Rest: 30–90 seconds between sets

Starting position: Stand up straight with your feet placed slightly wider than your hips. Turn your legs outward from the hip as far as is comfortable, keeping your knees, ankles, and toes aligned. Cross your hands at your chest, holding a weight in each hand or cradling the Body Bar.

Movement: Bend your knees, stopping when your knees directly align over your ankles. Return to the starting position.

Tips and techniques:
- Keep your torso upright and shoulders down and back.
- Squeeze your inner thighs as you straighten your legs to return to the starting position.
- Exhale as you lift up.

Too hard? Do the plié without weights, or bend your knees less as you plié.
Too easy? Use heavier weights.

Split strength workout: Upper body

These eight exercises will buff your upper body and make hauling the groceries—or powering your kayak through the water, making that shot down the fairway, or smashing an overhead in tennis—much easier. For a full strength routine, pair these upper-body exercises with the lower-body exercises in the previous workout. You can blend all of the exercises into a single workout or do the upper body one day and the lower body on another. A sturdy chair can substitute for a padded weight bench, and hand weights serve the same purpose as a Body Bar. Rest 48 hours between upper-body strength sessions, and bracket your workout with a warm-up and cool-down.

Equipment:
• Stability ball • Weight bench or sturdy chair • Weights • Body Bar (optional) • Mat, towels, or carpet for comfort during floor exercises

1 | Bent-over row

Reps: 8–12 on each side
Sets: 1–3
Intensity: Light to moderate
Tempo: 3-1
Rest: 30–90 seconds between sets

Starting position: Stand with a weight in your right hand and a bench or sturdy chair at your left side. Place your left hand and knee on the bench or chair seat and position your right hand directly under your right shoulder, fully extended toward the floor. Your spine should be neutral and your shoulders and hips squared.

Movement: Squeeze your shoulder blades together, then bend your elbow to slowly lift the weight toward your ribs. Return to the starting position. Finish all reps before repeating on the left side. This is one complete set.

Tips and techniques:
• Keep your shoulders squared throughout.
• Keep your elbow close to your side as you lift the weight.
• Exhale as you lift.

Too hard? Use a lighter weight.
Too easy? Use a heavier weight.

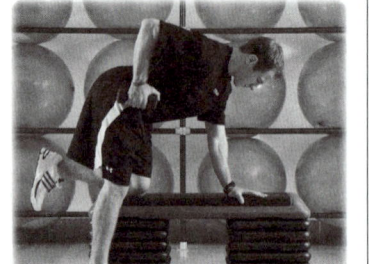

2 | V-raise

Reps: 8–12
Sets: 1–3
Intensity: Moderate
Tempo: 3-1-3
Rest: 30–90 seconds between sets

Starting position: Stand up straight holding weights at your sides with thumbs pointing forward. Lift your chest and roll your shoulders down and back.

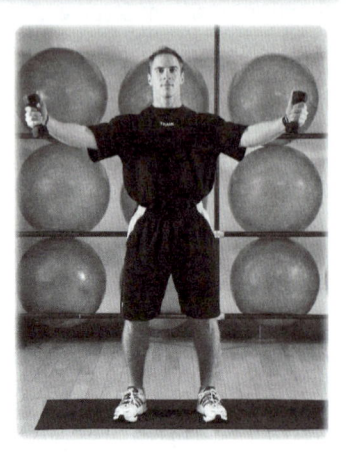

Movement: Squeeze your shoulder blades together as you slowly lift your arms toward the two front corners of the room, creating a "V" as you raise the weights. Go no higher than your shoulders. Pause, then return to the starting position.

Tips and techniques:
• Keep your thumbs pointing up throughout and your posture neutral with shoulders down and back.
• Keep your wrists firm, maintaining a straight line from your elbow to your knuckles, and elbows soft (not locked).
• Exhale as you lift.

Too hard? Use a lighter weight.
Too easy? Use a heavier weight.

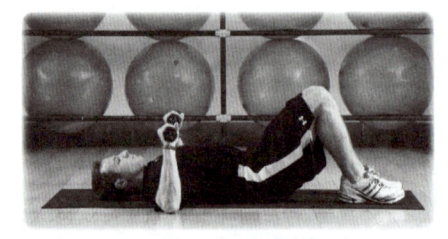

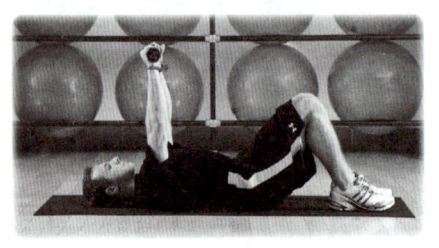

3 | Chest press

Reps: 8–12
Sets: 1–3
Intensity: Moderate
Tempo: 2-2
Rest: 30–90 seconds between sets

Starting position: Lie on your back on the floor, holding a weight in each hand, with your knees bent and feet flat, hip-width apart. Extend your arms straight over your chest toward the ceiling, palms facing the front wall. Keep your wrists firm and straight (like a metal pipe).

Movement: Tighten your abdominal muscles and keep your shoulder blades pressing into the floor as you bend your elbows to lower the weights, keeping your elbows in line with your shoulders. Return to the starting position.

Tips and techniques:
• Maintain core stability by tightening your abdominal muscles throughout the exercise.
• Exhale as you press up.

Too hard? Use lighter weights.
Too easy? Do the exercise in a bridge position on a stability ball, or use heavier weights.

38 Workout Workbook www.health.harvard.edu

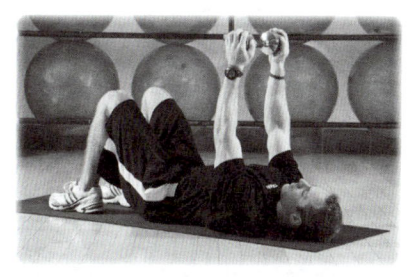

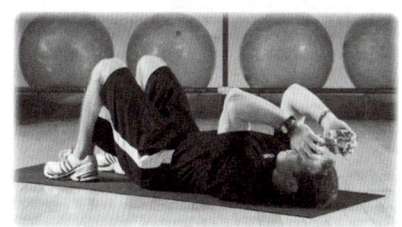

Split strength workout: Upper body

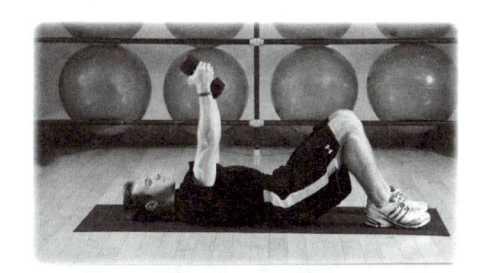

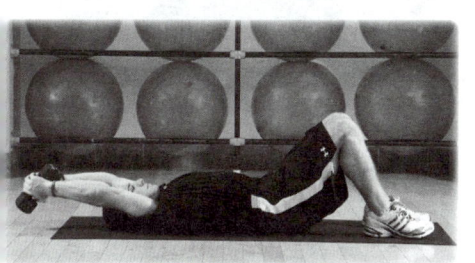

4 | Pull-over

Reps: 8–12
Sets: 1–3
Intensity: Moderate
Tempo: 4-1-4
Rest: 30–90 seconds after each set

Starting position: Lie on your back on the floor with your knees bent and feet flat, hip-width apart. Wrap both hands around the center of a single weight with thumbs pointing up. Extend your arms straight up over your chest.

Movement: Slowly lower the weight over your head toward the floor until your arms line up with your ears. Pause, then tighten your abdominal muscles as you lift the weight back to the starting position.

Tips and techniques:
- Keep your wrists firm and in line with your elbows as you hold the weight.
- Before lowering your weight overhead, press your shoulder blades down and back into the floor to stabilize your shoulders.
- Exhale as you lift up.

Too hard? Use a lighter weight.
Too easy? Use a heavier weight.

5 | Chest fly

Reps: 8–12
Sets: 1–3
Intensity: Moderate
Tempo: 2-2
Rest: 30–90 seconds between sets

Starting position: Lie on your back on the floor with your knees bent and feet flat, hip-width apart. Hold weights with your palms facing each other, and extend your arms toward the ceiling directly over your chest.

Movement: Contract your abdominal muscles and press your shoulder blades back into the floor. Slowly lower your arms out to each side, stopping just above the floor. Focus on using your chest muscles while lifting the weights back to the starting position over your chest.

Tips and techniques:
- As you lower your arms, keep your elbows slightly relaxed so that the joints aren't overextended.
- Control the weights throughout the exercise, keeping your shoulders and torso stable.
- Exhale as you lift.

Too hard? Use lighter weights.
Too easy? Use heavier weights.

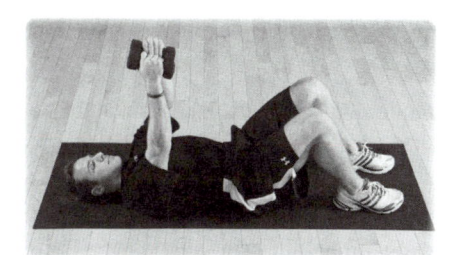

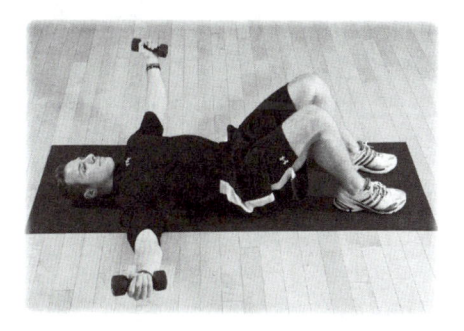

6 | Triceps press

Reps: 8–12
Sets: 1–3
Intensity: Light to moderate
Tempo: 3-1
Rest: 30–90 seconds between sets

Starting position: Lie on your back on the floor with your knees bent and feet flat, hip-width apart. Hold one weight at both of its ends with your palms facing each other. Extend your arms toward the ceiling directly in line over your shoulders.

Movement: Holding your wrists firm, slowly bend your elbows and lower the weight toward the top of your head. Exhale as you return to starting position.

Tips and techniques:
- Keep your elbows directly in line with your shoulders throughout.
- Keep your shoulders down and back.
- As you lower the weight toward the top of your head, keep your elbows pointing toward the ceiling.

Too hard? Use a lighter weight.
Too easy? Use a heavier weight.

Split strength workout: Upper body

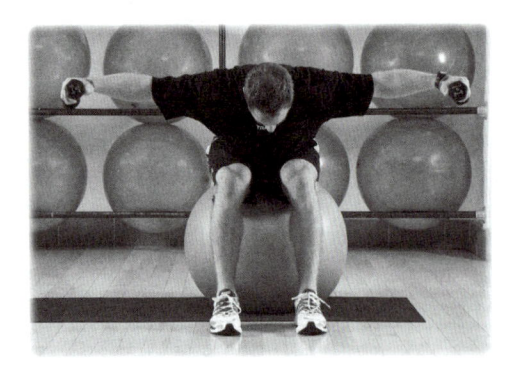

7 | Back fly

Reps: 8–12
Sets: 1–3
Intensity: Moderate
Tempo: 2-1-2
Rest: 30–90 seconds between sets

Starting position: Sit on a stability ball, holding weights at your sides with your palms facing toward your body and thumbs pointing forward. Hinge forward from your hips, bringing your chest toward your thighs.

Movement: Squeeze your shoulder blades together, then slowly lift the weights out to the sides until your arms are about shoulder height. Keep your elbows soft, not locked. Pause, then return to the starting position.

Tips and techniques:

- Throughout the movement, squeeze your shoulder blades together.
- Control the movement without using any momentum.
- Exhale as you lift.

Too hard? Use lighter weights or no weights.
Too easy? Use heavier weights.

8 | Concentrated biceps curl

Reps: 8–12 on each side
Sets: 1–3
Intensity: Moderate to high
Tempo: 3-1-3
Rest: 30–90 seconds between sets

Starting position: Sit on a stability ball or weight bench, feet hip-width apart, holding a weight in your right hand. Hinge forward slightly from your hips and anchor the elbow of your right arm inside your right inner thigh near the knee. Fully extend your arm, thumb pointing forward, so the weight comes down toward the floor, while keeping your elbow soft.

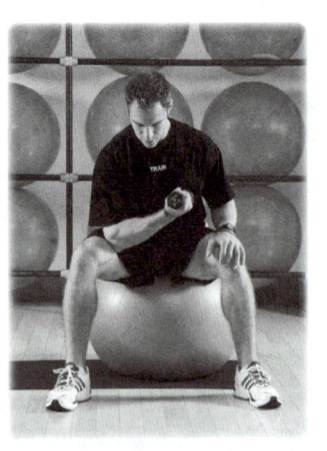

Movement: Keeping your shoulders down and back, bend your right arm at the elbow to raise the weight toward your right shoulder. Pause, then slowly lower to the starting position. Finish all reps before repeating with your left arm. This is one complete set.

Tips and techniques:

- Be careful not to lock your elbow (hyperextension) as you straighten your arm to return to the starting position.
- Keep your torso and your shoulders still throughout.
- Exhale as you lift.

Too hard? Use a lighter weight.
Too easy? Use a heavier weight.

SUPERSET ME

Want to try supersets? Combine these:
- Bent-over row + V-raise
- Pull-over + Chest fly

See "Supersets," page 17, for more information.

Power challenge workout

Strength helps you stroll to your bus stop. Power pushes you into a sweat-popping sprint on the final block so you catch that bus before the doors close. The explosive moves in this tough, challenging workout—including plyometric jumps that imitate moves used in different sports—require you to pour on power and strength. Meanwhile, the Bosu works your core and enhances stability, while jumping rope between each exercise pumps up your cardiovascular system, too. Remember to bracket your workout with a warm-up and cool-down.

Equipment:
- Jump rope
- Medicine ball (optional)

1 | Forward jump onto Bosu

Reps: 8–12
Sets: 1–3
Intensity: Moderate to high
Tempo: 2-2
Rest: 30–90 seconds between sets

Starting position: Stand up straight in front of a Bosu with your feet slightly apart and your arms at your sides.

Movement: Slightly bend both knees to gather energy, then jump up onto the Bosu, landing with both feet slightly apart while bending your elbows to bring your hands up toward your chest. Step back off the Bosu one foot at a time to return to the starting position.

Tips and techniques:
- Tighten your abdominal muscles and lean forward slightly from the hips, keeping a straight line from the top of your head to your tailbone to help propel your body forward.
- Alternate the lead foot as you step down from the Bosu.

Too hard? Step up onto the Bosu one foot at a time. Pause, then step down one foot at a time.
Too easy? After jumping up onto the Bosu, add an extra small jump on the top, before stepping back down.

2 | Jump rope

Reps: 1–2 minutes
Sets: 1 set *between* each of the Power Challenge exercises
Intensity: High
Tempo: Set your own pace
Rest: 30–90 seconds before moving to the next exercise

Starting position: Stand up straight, holding the jump rope behind you in the ready position.

Movement: Jump rope with both feet, or do one foot at a time.

Tips and techniques:
- Maintain neutral posture with shoulders relaxed, down, and back.
- Remember to breathe!

Too hard? Do the jump-rope action without the rope.
Too easy? Increase your jumping speed.

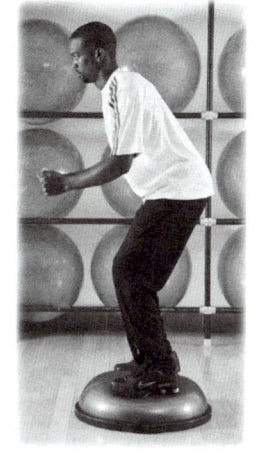

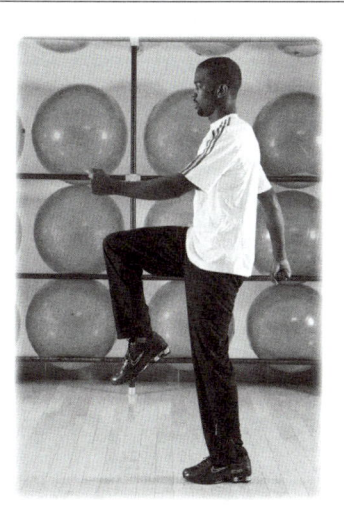

3 | Walking knee lift with hop

Reps: 8–12
Sets: 1–3
Intensity: Moderate to high
Tempo: 1-1
Rest: 30–90 seconds between sets

Starting position: Stand up straight with your feet a few inches apart.

Movement: Step forward with your right foot. As you do a knee lift with the left leg, hop on your right foot, letting your arms swing naturally. Now step forward on your left foot as you do a knee lift with the right leg and hop on your left foot, letting your arms swing naturally.

Tips and techniques:
- Stand up straight and tighten your abdominal muscles throughout.
- Think of lengthening your body as you hop straight up.

Too hard? Do as a walking knee lift without the hop.
Too easy? As you do the hop, lift your arms up high overhead.

Power challenge workout

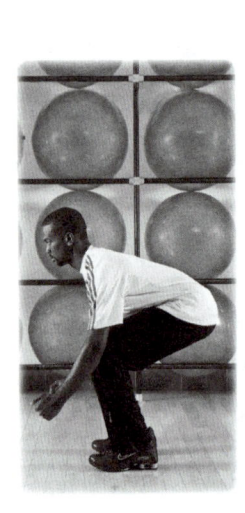

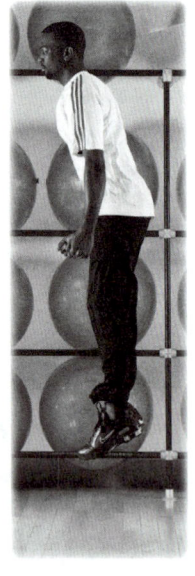

4 | Squat with jump

Reps: 8–12
Sets: 1–3
Intensity: Moderate to high
Tempo: 1-1
Rest: 30–90 seconds between sets

Starting position: Stand with your feet shoulder-width apart and your arms down at your sides. Hinge forward at the hips and bend your knees in a squat position. Try to keep your knees vertically aligned over your ankles. Tighten your abdominal muscles and keep your shoulders down and back.

Movement: Jump up, straightening your legs, and land on both feet in the starting position. Repeat until you complete all reps.

Tips and techniques:

- Sit back in the squat position as if sitting in a chair, pressing your weight back into your heels.
- Keep your hips, knees, ankles, and toes pointing forward, and your head and neck in line with your spine.
- Land softly on both feet.

Too hard? From the squat position, straighten your legs without jumping and then return to bent knees.
Too easy? As you jump, extend your arms overhead, or hold a medicine ball.

5 | Alternating lunge with jump

Reps: 8–12
Sets: 1–3
Intensity: Moderate to high
Tempo: 1-1
Rest: 30–90 seconds between sets

Starting position: Stand in the lunge position with the right foot forward and left foot back. Your right knee should align over the ankle, and your left knee should point to the floor. Place your hands at your sides.

Movement: From the lunge position, jump straight up and change legs before landing. Repeat with the left foot forward and right foot back for one full rep. Continue to alternate legs to complete all reps.

Tips and techniques:

- In the lunge position, keep your abdominal muscles tightened, your shoulders down and back, and your hips, knees, ankles, and feet all facing forward.
- The knee of your back leg should point to the floor, and your front knee should not extend beyond the arch of the supporting foot.

Too hard? Do alternating lunges without the jump.
Too easy? Extend your arms out to the side as you do the exercise.

6 | Squat shuffle

Reps: 8–12
Sets: 1–3
Intensity: Moderate to high
Tempo: 1-1
Rest: 30–90 seconds between sets

Starting position: Stand up straight with your feet comfortably together and your hands by your sides.

Movement: Step to the right into a squat, bending your elbows to bring your hands up with palms forward, then bring your left foot in to your right foot while staying in the squat position. Do 4–6 of these traveling "squat shuffles" to the right, then immediately do 4–6 squat shuffles to the left.

Tips and techniques:

- Maintain control and correct alignment throughout: slightly sitting back, straight line from top of head to tailbone, shoulders down and back.
- Remember to breathe!

Too hard? Do traveling squats to the side at a slower pace.
Too easy? Increase speed, or hold a medicine ball.

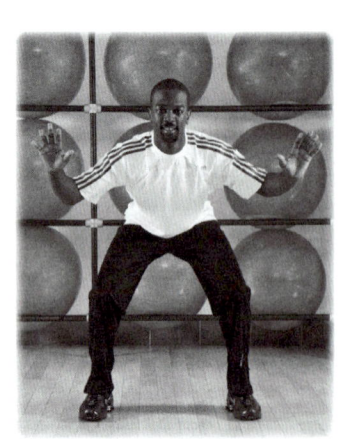

Power challenge workout

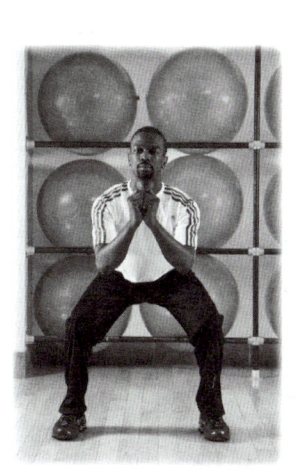

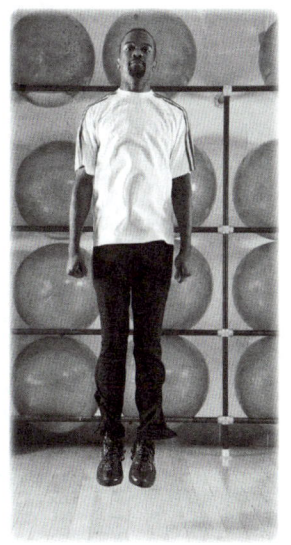

7 | Side-to-side squat press

Reps: Follow the sequence below
Sets: 1–3
Intensity: Moderate to high
Tempo: See pattern under "Movement," below
Rest: 30–90 seconds between sets

Starting position: Stand up straight with your feet comfortably together, and bend your elbows to bring your hands up toward your chest.

Movement: Step out to the side with your right foot, into a squat. Stay in this position and pulse, pressing down slightly, for 8 counts. From the squat position, do a small jump to straighten up and bring your feet together, letting your hands fall to your sides. Then raise your hands again as you bring your left foot out to the side for the squat. Pulse 8 counts again and do a small jump to bring your feet together. Repeat on your right foot, pulse 4 counts. Repeat on your left foot, pulse 4 counts. Repeat on your right foot, pulse 2 counts. Repeat on your left foot, pulse 2 counts. Then do single counts, alternating right and left legs on the squat, for 2–6 more reps. This is one complete set.

Tips and techniques:
- Remember the correct squat position throughout: slightly sitting back, straight line from top of head to tailbone, shoulders down and back.
- Distribute weight evenly between both feet as you squat from side to side.
- Remember to breathe!

Too hard? When doing side squats, bring your feet together without the jump. Also, limit reps by doing only the 8 pulses before switching legs, then resting.
Too easy? Each time you change the lead foot, lift it up on the jump.

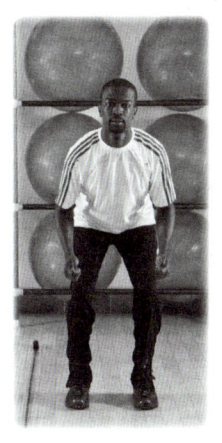

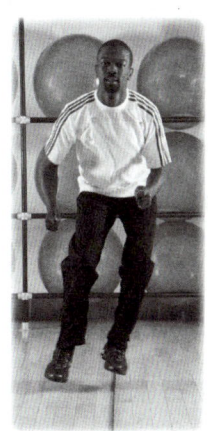

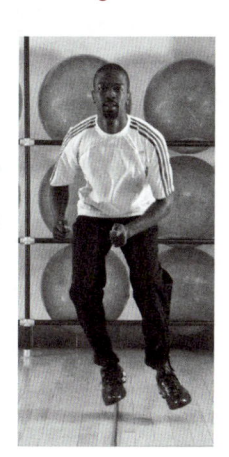

8 | Lateral jump

Reps: 8–12
Sets: 1–3
Intensity: Moderate to high
Tempo: 1-1-1
Rest: 30–90 seconds between sets

Starting position: Stand up straight to the left of a jump rope stretched out on the floor. Place your arms comfortably at your sides.

Movement: Slightly bend knees to gather energy. Then jump to the right with both feet, going up and over the outstretched rope while bending your elbows to bring your hands toward your chest. Land on both feet at the same time with knees slightly bent. Pause, then jump over the rope to the left.

Tips and techniques:
- Maintain a neutral spine, keeping your shoulders down and back.
- Keep your hips, knees, ankles, and toes all pointing forward.
- Exhale as you jump to the side.

Too hard? Sidestep to the right, then quickly bring the left foot together with the right foot. Repeat to the other side.
Too easy? Jump over a step placed lengthwise at your right side.

Complex challenge workout

Complex workouts blend two or three distinct exercises into one. That cranks up your workout considerably. Just six exercises offer a challenging full-body workout. Control is key! Perform each exercise slowly and with great concentration, using lighter weights than usual at first, if need be. Bracket your workout with a warm-up and cool-down.

Equipment:
- Stability ball • Weights
- Mat, towels, or carpet for comfort during floor exercises

1 | Chest fly and chest press on stability ball

Sets: 1–3
Intensity: Moderate
Tempo: 2-2
Rest: 30–90 seconds between sets

Starting position: Sit on the stability ball holding a weight in each hand. Roll downward until the back of your head and shoulders are on the stability ball. Position your feet shoulder-width apart and lift your hips and buttocks up in the bridge position. Align your knees directly over your ankles. Extend your arms toward the ceiling, with palms facing each other.

Movement: *For the chest fly:* Tighten your abdominal muscles. Press your shoulder blades back into the ball as you slowly lower your arms straight out to the sides no farther than shoulder level. Keep your shoulders and torso still while lifting the weights back to the starting position over your chest.

For the chest press: Rotate your extended arms so that your palms are facing in the direction of your feet. Bend your elbows out to the side in line with your shoulders as you bring the weights down, being careful not to let your elbows go lower than the stability ball. Press upward to return to the starting position.

First set: Do chest fly 8–12 times, chest press 8–12 times.

Second set: Do chest fly 4–6 times, chest press 4–6 times. Repeat once.

Third set: Do chest fly, then chest press. Repeat combination 8–12 times.

Tips and techniques:
- Tighten your abdominal and buttock muscles to maintain stability and alignment in shoulders, hips, knees, ankles, and feet.
- Choose weights heavy enough to challenge you during the repetitions, but light enough to allow you to stay in control and go through a full range of motion. This is especially important when alternating chest fly and chest press.

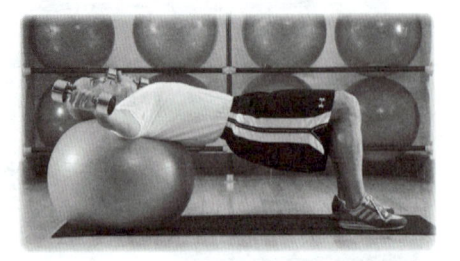

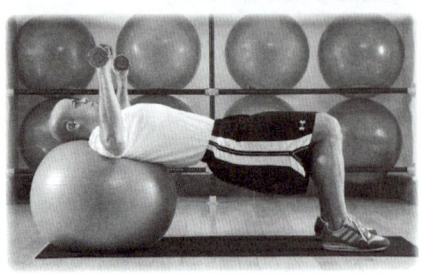

Too hard? Use lighter weights and do fewer repetitions, or do the exercises while lying on the floor.
Too easy? Use heavier weights.

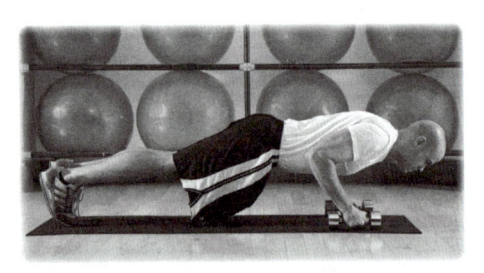

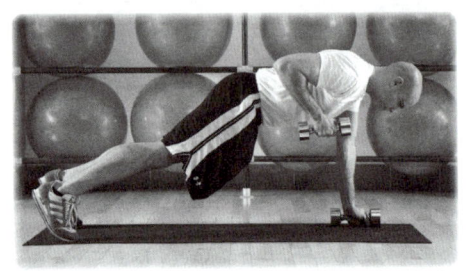

2 | Push-up and alternating row

Sets: 1–3
Intensity: Moderate to high
Tempo: 2-2
Rest: 30–90 seconds between sets

Starting position: Position yourself at the top of a push-up with your arms straight and directly under your shoulders, hands resting on dumbbells, legs extended, and feet flexed with toes touching the floor. Tighten your abdominal muscles to help maintain a neutral spine so your body aligns from the top of your head to your heels.

Movement: *For the push-up:* Keep your abdominal muscles tightened and maintain a neutral spine as you bend your arms to lower your chest toward the floor. Push up to return to the starting position.

For the alternating row: Stay in the push-up position as you pull the right weight up toward your chest until your hand is close to your rib cage. Lower the weight and repeat on the left side.

First set: Do 8–12 push-ups, 8–12 alternating rows.

Second set: Do 4–6 push-ups, 4–6 alternating rows. Repeat combination once.

Third set: Do 2 push-ups, 2 alternating rows. Repeat combination 3–5 times.

Tips and techniques:
- Keep your head and spine neutral.
- Lead with your chest (not head) as you lower yourself into the push-up.
- Inhale as you lower; exhale as you lift.

Too hard? Perform the push-ups with your knees on the floor.
Too easy? Use heavier weights.

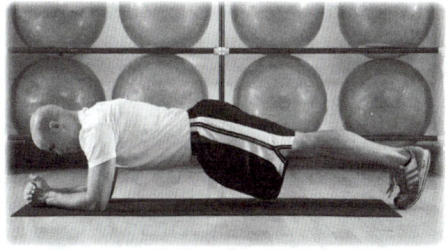

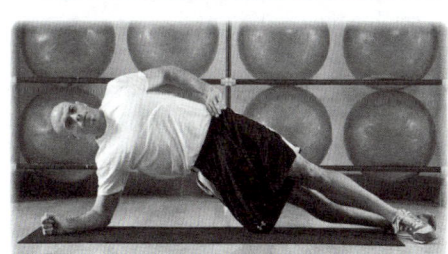

Complex challenge workout

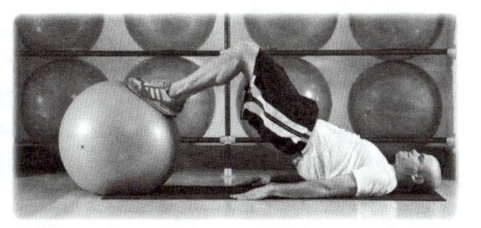

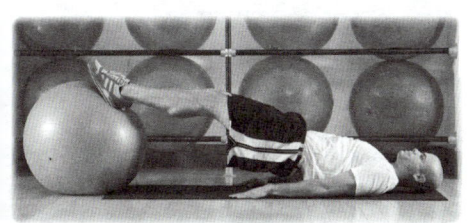

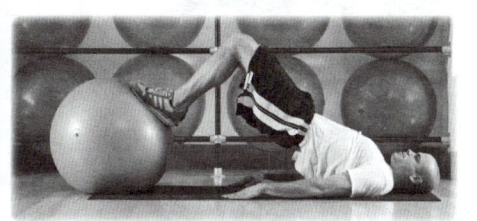

3 | Bridge, leg extension, and hamstring curl

Sets: 1–3
Intensity: Moderate to high
Tempo: 2-2-2-2
Rest: 30–90 seconds between sets

Starting position: Lie on your back on the floor with your knees bent and feet flat on the upper side of a stability ball. Put your hands down at your sides on the floor.

Movement: *For the bridge:* Squeeze your buttocks while lifting your hips by pressing your feet into the ball.
For the leg extension: Keeping your core still and stable, straighten your legs to roll the ball away from you.
For the hamstring curl: Pull the ball back toward you by bending your knees in a hamstring curl. Lower your hips back to the floor to return to the starting position.
First set: Repeat the combination of bridge, leg extension, and hamstring curl 8–12 times.
Second set: Squeeze your buttocks while lifting your hips in the bridge. Perform a leg extension followed by a hamstring curl 4 times before lowering your hips to the floor. Repeat 2–3 times.
Third set: Squeeze your buttocks while lifting your hips in the bridge. Perform a leg extension followed by a hamstring curl 8–12 times before lowering your hips to the floor.

Tips and techniques:
- Keep your spine neutral and avoid arching your back.
- Avoid locking your knees as you extend your legs on the ball.

Too hard? Do the bridge, then lower your hips to the floor for the leg extension and hamstring curl.
Too easy? Try lifting your arms off the floor or bringing them across your chest.

4 | Front plank and side plank

Sets: 1–3
Intensity: Moderate to high
Tempo: See below
Rest: 30–90 seconds between sets

Starting position: Start on your hands and knees.

Movement: *For the front plank:* Tighten your abdominal muscles and lower your upper body so your forearms are on the floor, with hands clasped, aligning your shoulders directly over your elbows. Extend both legs with your feet flexed and toes touching the floor so that you balance your body in a line like a plank. Hold for 8 counts, then move to the side plank.
For the side plank: Turn your whole body so your left side is upward and you balance on your right forearm and the inside of your left foot, which should be positioned slightly in front of the outside of your right foot. Nothing between these points should touch the floor. Keep your shoulders and hips in a straight line and rest your left hand on your left hip. Hold 8 counts.
Return to the front plank and hold 8 counts. Then turn your whole body in the other direction so that you balance on your left forearm and the inside of your right foot, positioned slightly in front of the outside of your left foot. Hold 8 more counts.
First set: Hold 8 counts during the front plank, right side plank, front plank, left side plank.
Second set: Hold 6 counts during the front plank, right side plank, front plank, left side plank. Repeat sequence 2 times.
Third set: Hold 4 counts during the front plank, right side plank, front plank, left side plank. Repeat sequence 4 times.

Tips and techniques:
- Always maintain a neutral spine.
- Stay in control throughout the movement.
- Breathe comfortably.

Too hard? Lower your knees to the ground in each position.
Too easy? Hold longer in each position.

Complex challenge workout

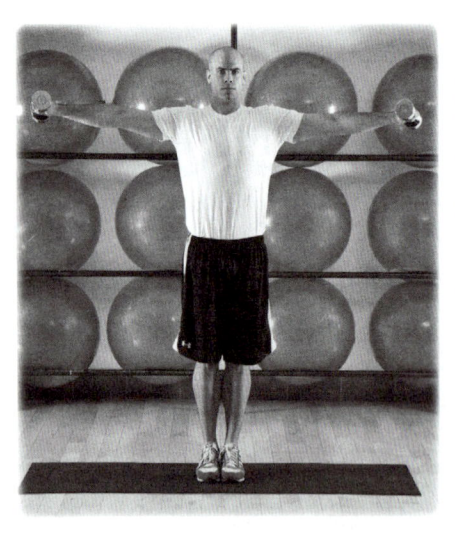

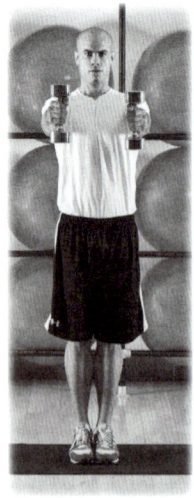

5 | Lateral raise and front raise

Sets: 1–3
Intensity: Moderate
Tempo: 2-1-2
Rest: 30–90 seconds between sets

Starting position: Stand up straight with your hands at your sides holding weights. Keep your thumbs pointing forward.

Movement: *For the lateral raise:* Tighten your abdominal, buttock, and mid-back muscles as you raise your arms straight out to the side, no higher than shoulder level. Pause, then lower to the starting position.

For the front raise: Raise both arms forward no higher than shoulder level with your thumbs up. Pause, then lower to the starting position.

First set: Do 8–12 lateral raises, 8–12 front raises.

Second set: Do 1 lateral raise, then 1 front raise. Repeat combination 8–12 times.

Third set: Lift the right arm to the side for a lateral raise as you simultaneously lift your left arm forward for a front raise. Pause, then lower both arms to the starting position. Repeat, doing a lateral raise with your left arm and front raise with your right arm. Repeat combination 8–12 times.

Tips and techniques:
• Keep your shoulders, hips, knees, and ankles still and facing front throughout.
• Control the lateral lifts and front raises so you perform them without relying on momentum.
• Exhale as you lift.

Too hard? Do fewer repetitions using lighter weights. Do only the first and second sets.
Too easy? Use heavier weights.

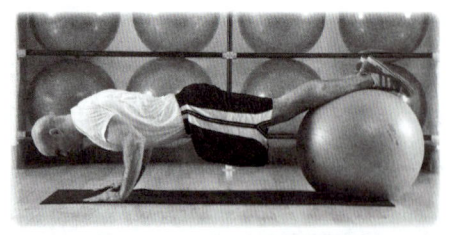

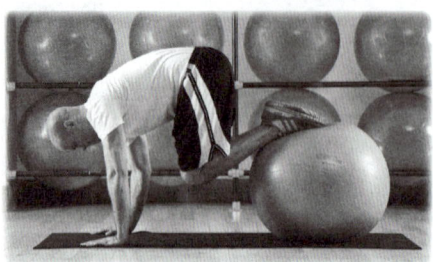

6 | Push-up and abdominal curl on stability ball

Sets: 1–3
Intensity: Moderate to high
Tempo: 2-1-2
Rest: 30–90 seconds between sets

Starting position: Lie on your stomach with your thighs on a stability ball and hands on the floor. Walk your hands out, letting the ball roll along your legs, until you are in a comfortable plank position, keeping your hands directly under your shoulders and tightening your abdominal muscles.

Movement: *For the push-up:* Bend your elbows to lower your chest toward the floor. Pause, then extend your arms to return to the plank position.

For the abdominal curl: Starting in the plank position, use your abdominal and leg muscles as you bend your knees to draw the ball in toward your chest. Pause, then stabilize your core as you extend your legs to push the ball back and return to the plank position.

First set: Do 8–12 push-ups, 8–12 abdominal curls.

Second set: Do 2 push-ups, then 2 abdominal curls. Repeat 3–5 times.

Third set: Do 1 push-up, then 1 abdominal curl. Repeat combination 8–12 times.

Tips and techniques:
• Keep your abdominal muscles tightened and your core stationary throughout the exercise.
• Keep your shoulders down and back.

Too hard? Walk your hands out a shorter distance from the ball before doing push-ups and curls.
Too easy? While maintaining correct alignment with your hands directly under your shoulders, walk your hands farther away from the ball before doing push-ups and curls.

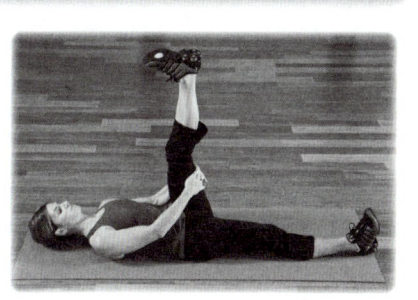

Cool-down

After a workout, cooling down for five to 10 minutes through a sequence of slow movements helps prevent muscle cramps and dizziness while slowing quick breathing and a fast-beating heart. Our cool-down enhances flexibility by stretching muscles throughout your body and mixes in calming yoga moves. Flow from one movement to another without rests in between. You'll achieve best results by holding stretches for 10 to 30 seconds and doing these exercises at least two or three times a week. The longer you can hold a stretch, the better for flexibility.

Equipment:
- Mat, towels, or carpet for comfort during floor exercises

1 | Torso rotation

Reps: 4
Sets: 1
Intensity: Light
Hold: 10–30 seconds

Starting position: Lie on your back with your knees bent and feet together flat on the floor. Put your arms comfortably out to each side just below shoulder level, palms up.

Movement: Tighten your abdominal muscles as you lower both knees together toward one side of the floor. Keeping your shoulders still and flat on the floor, look in the opposite direction. Feel the stretch across your chest and torso. Hold. Return to the starting position. Repeat in the opposite direction.

Tips and techniques:
- Stretch to the point of mild tension.
- Keep your shoulders relaxed and pressing into the floor.
- Breathe comfortably.

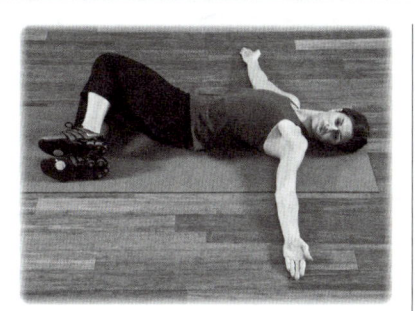

2 | Hamstring stretch

Reps: 4 on each side
Sets: 1
Intensity: Light
Hold: 10–30 seconds

Starting position: Lie on your back with your right leg extended on the floor. Hold your left leg with both hands behind the thigh so your knee is bent and directly above your hip.

Movement: Flex the foot of the bent left leg and lift the heel toward the ceiling, straightening the leg as much as possible without locking the knee. As you do so, flex the foot on your extended right leg to stretch the calf muscles and the hip flexor at the front of the hip, a spot that is tight in many people. Hold. Return to the starting position. Finish all reps before repeating with the leg positions reversed. This is one complete set.

Tips and techniques:
- Stretch the leg extended toward the ceiling to the point of mild tension without any pressure behind the knee.
- Breathe comfortably.

3 | Upper hip stretch

Reps: 4
Sets: 1
Intensity: Light
Hold: 10–30 seconds

Starting position: Lie on your back with your right knee bent and your foot on the floor. Rest your left ankle on your right kneecap. Your left knee should point toward the side. Hold the back of the right thigh with both hands.

Movement: Relax your shoulders down and back as you lift your right foot up off the floor until you feel tightness in your left hip and buttock. Hold. Return to the starting position. Repeat on the opposite side.

Tips and techniques:
- Stretch to the point of mild tension.
- Hold the stretch as still as possible without bouncing.
- Breathe comfortably.

4 | Upward dog

Reps: 4 **Sets:** 1
Intensity: Light
Hold: 10–30 seconds

Starting position: Lie on your stomach with your hands next to your shoulders, palms facing down, and legs comfortably extended.

Movement: Slowly lift your head, shoulders, and chest off the floor by pressing your palms against the floor. Keep your head and neck in neutral alignment as you try to fully straighten your arms. Hold. Return slowly to the starting position.

Tips and techniques:
- Lift only to the point of mild tension.
- Be careful not to lock your elbows while fully straightening your arms.
- Breathe comfortably, or practice yoga breathing.

Cool-down

5 | Child's pose with diagonal reach

Reps: 4
Sets: 1
Intensity: Light
Hold: 10–30 seconds

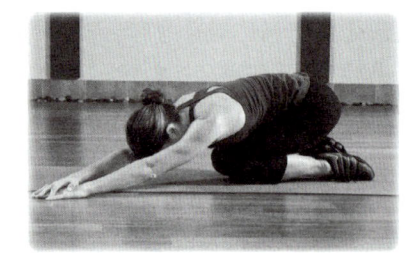

Starting position: Start on your hands and knees. Walk your hands diagonally out to the right and place your left hand on top of your right hand. Keep your shoulders down and back as you do so.

Movement: Slowly drop your buttocks back toward your heels. Hold. Return to the starting position. Repeat on the opposite side.

Tips and techniques:
- Stretch to the point of mild tension.
- Breathe comfortably.

6 | Downward-facing dog

Reps: 4
Sets: 1
Intensity: Light to moderate
Hold: 10–30 seconds

Starting position: Start on your hands and knees.

Movement: Lift your knees off the floor until your legs extend so you are in an upside-down "V," aligning your ears and arms while maintaining a neutral neck and spine. Try to keep your weight evenly distributed between hands and feet. If possible, press your heels toward the floor. Keep your shoulders down and back. Hold. Return to the starting position.

Tips and techniques:
- Think of lengthening your spine as you engage your abdominal muscles.
- Breathe comfortably, or practice yoga breathing if you've been taught this.

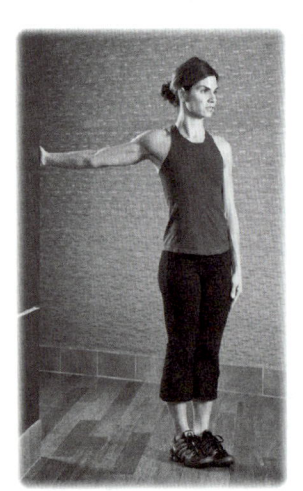

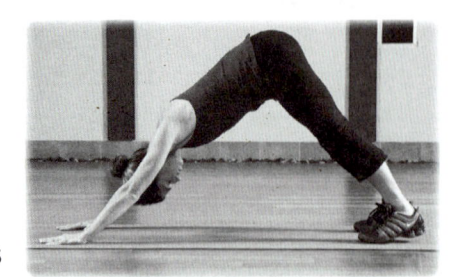

7 | Chest stretch

Reps: 4 on each side
Sets: 1
Intensity: Light to moderate
Hold: 10–30 seconds

Starting position: Stand in a doorway facing forward. Put your right hand on the edge of the door frame slightly below shoulder level, palm facing forward. Keep your shoulders down and back.

Movement: Slowly turn your body to the left, away from the door frame, until you feel the stretch in your chest and shoulder. Hold. Finish all reps before repeating on the opposite side. This is one complete set.

Tips and techniques:
- Stretch to the point of mild tension.
- Breathe comfortably.

8 | Shoulder stretch with torso rotation

Reps: 4 on each side
Sets: 1
Intensity: Light
Hold: 10–30 seconds

Starting position: Stand with your feet hip-width apart. Put your left hand on your right shoulder. Cup your left elbow with your right hand.

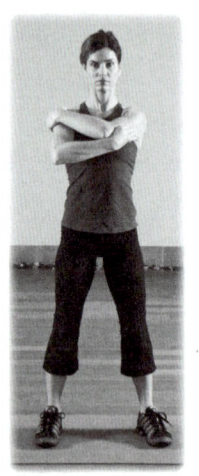

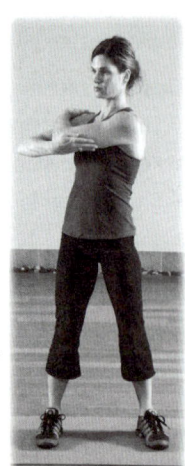

Movement: Roll your shoulders down and back as you gently pull your left elbow across your chest.

Pause, then rotate your torso to the right while keeping your hips, knees, and feet facing forward. Hold. Return to the starting position. Finish all reps before repeating on the other side.

Tips and techniques:
- Keep your shoulders down and back.
- Stretch to the point of mild tension.
- Breathe comfortably.